When Your Parent Becomes Your Child:

Advice for Caregivers

…from a Daughter Who Spent 23 Years

Dealing with Aging and Dementia

ISBN 978-1-60910-741-3

Library of Congress Control Number: 2011902989

Printed in the United States of America on acid-free paper.
Published in the United States by Booklocker.com, Inc.,
Bangor, Maine, 2011. First Edition

The content of this book is for informational use only and is not intended to replace professional medical or legal advice.

Cover Photograph:
The author's parents, George & Violette Tarnow, on their wedding day, April 4, 1931, taken by Violette's brother, WALTER SCHOEN.

Cover Illustrations:
Dove and heart drawn by Mr. & Mrs. Tarnow's great-grandson, ETHAN C. LAPITAN. For more information, visit Ethan at www.Ethan.ws.

Cover Design:
TODD ENGEL

When Your Parent Becomes Your Child: Advice for Caregivers
…from a Daughter Who Spent 23 Years Dealing with Aging and Dementia

Georgette H. Tarnow

Booklocker.com, Inc., Bangor, ME

First Edition

DEDICATION

To all the caregivers who give of themselves to help others
lead better lives.

To all my friends and relatives who supported me through both my
caregiving and my writing, especially my aunt, RUTH TARNOW CATO, for
her faith.

This book would not have been possible if my dear, beloved cousin,
ROSE MARIE DITTO GRASS, had not insisted to me,
"Write it down!"

ABOUT THE AUTHOR

GEORGETTE H. TARNOW, JD, LLM, is an attorney and author who spent 23 years as a full-time caregiver for her parents. Ms. Tarnow was praised by doctors and various health care professionals for her common sense approach and understanding of the needs of the elderly. Her articles have appeared in numerous publications and she also blogs about caregiving. She may be reached at Info@YourCaregiving.com.

Ms. Tarnow's website, www.YourCaregiving.com, is dedicated to assisting caregivers and to preserving the dignity of the elderly and victims of dementia. *When Your Parent Becomes Your Child* is the first of several books by Ms. Tarnow for YourCaregiving.com.

ACKNOWLEDGMENTS

Thanks to my copy editor, KATHLEEN BIGNESS-BEDRIO, for her editing assistance and empathy. Any errors are mine.

A special thank you to author TOM WOLFERMAN (www.tomwolferman.com) for allowing me to use an excerpt from *Prairie Dogs Are Contagious*, one of a series of caregiving essays, in Chapter Seven—Humor.

My mother was a terrific storyteller. Because of her poor eyesight, she never read to me but she made up stories to tell me. A brief excerpt of one of her tales, *Pink Curls: A Christmas Story*, appears here in Chapter Six—Paranoia. Please visit www.PinkCurls.com for more information.

TABLE OF CONTENTS

PREFACE

Cast me not off in the time of old age; forsake me not when my strength faileth.

-Psalms 71:9 (King James Version)

DIVORCE WAS ALMOST unheard of during the World War I era, but both my grandparents on my mother's side and my father's side divorced during that period.

My father, George J. Tarnow, born in 1907, was the elder of two children. Around 1915, his father abandoned the family. His mother went outside the home to work finding whatever jobs she could. For a while, she worked in Sears' shipping department, wrapping the mail orders. That meant Dad had many chores around the house. Hard things like carrying up the buckets of coal to the third floor apartment. Dad was able to attend high school for two years before working full time. He became a lithographer, a sort of printer, and worked at that trade until his retirement at 62. He served in the Navy in World War II making naval charts in Washington, DC.

My mother, Violette Schoen Tarnow, born in 1911, was the youngest of seven children. Her father abandoned the family also around 1915. Her mother, having several young children, couldn't work outside the home. Mom was the lucky one: unlike her six siblings, she went to high school, if only for two years. Mom began working at 14 but didn't have to work full time until she was 16. She became a secretary but stopped working when she married Dad.

My parents met at a Chicago amusement park called Riverview, where they both worked part time. Mom was about 15, and wore costumes and rode on the floats in the nightly parades. Dad was about 18 and worked in the carpentry department. They married in 1931.

My mother began showing signs of what the doctors called senile dementia around 1978. She died in 1997 at the age of 86.

My father had a heart attack in 1991 and passed away in 2001 at the age of 93. Despite various ailments, he was quite spry to the end. His mental ability declined very little, although there were certain "quirks."

My parents were fortyish when I was born so I became a caregiver at an early age. I began caring for Mom when she first began showing signs of dementia and ended my career as a caregiver with my father's death. I spent 23 years as a live-in caregiver, staying with my parents in their home.

Together we dealt with heart disease, leukemia, arthritis, diabetes, enlarged prostate, prostate cancer, deafness, blindness, severe high blood pressure, and senile dementia.

This is our story.

INTRODUCTION

All sorrows can be borne if you put them into a story or tell a story about them.

-Isak Dinesen

THE FIRST TIME I ACTED as a caregiver was when my parents celebrated their wedding anniversary with a party at our house.

One of the guests was my Aunt Fanny (not her real name), my mother's sister. Fanny had had a mild stroke sometime previously but was functioning pretty well. However, when she went to our bathroom, she had a problem, so some of her urine wound up on the bathroom floor.

Mom asked me to clean up the bathroom. I did, but it wasn't easy and by the time I finished I was disheveled and sweaty. I can still remember the sweet, sick smell of her urine—I later learned she had diabetes. I wasn't happy to do the chore, but it had to be done. When I rejoined the party, Aunt Fanny loudly observed to me, "You look like hell!"

Well, yes, I suppose I did because it was a hot, dirty job cleaning up after her. That was my introduction to the world of caregiving. I was seven years old.

I'm not a doctor or nurse, although on several occasions when talking to doctors I was mistaken for a health care professional. My journey in caregiving led to learning a great deal about many diseases, drugs, and dementia. We were fortunate to have a family physician that made me his partner in caring for my parents.

I'm an attorney. My approach to law is as a sort of caregiver, as well. I specifically went to law school to help my extended family. I hated the notion that we could be threatened with lawsuits or become embroiled in any legal matter, and we would have to turn to a stranger for help.

We talked about caregiving in law school. I had a professor who cared for his senile father. He said we had a 50-50 chance of having to care for a parent with dementia. Little did I think then that I would be doing so within a year.

Why did I choose to be a caregiver? I don't think I ever consciously did. Being a caregiver is often not a role you choose--more likely it is something that happens to you; you are usually drafted and didn't enlist. Instead, I faced a long series of decisions and I "inadvertently" became a caregiver because of those choices.

When I was quite young one of my cynical friends said we should marry as soon as possible because any sibling who is unmarried when the parents need help becomes the caregiver until they die.

I was graduated from law school in 1980 and had every intention of working for the federal government, a good choice for women attorneys at that time. A government hiring freeze went into effect just as I was ready to enter the work force, though, so that was not an option. Job prospects in the private sector were rather dismal and became worse in 1981. Perhaps if I had been made the type of offer I couldn't refuse, such as a well-paid position with a law firm, my family's story would have been very different. As it was, I cared for my mother while I job hunted from home.

Maybe it was learned behavior. As a child, I was almost a daily visitor to the house where my mother grew up. Two of my aunts who never married shared this home with their mother, my grandmother, caring for her until the end.

Maybe it's what family does.

My dad swore Mother would never be put into a nursing home and I agreed with him. I personally believe if a healthy young person were to be put into a home, be over medicated, and be cut off from the outside world, that person would experience a mental decline. How much more so for the elderly person! My Aunt Min did go to a nursing home and had a positive experience. However, she was in a converted house with a very small group of patients. A devoted husband and wife team ran it.

I had two other aunts who needed care toward the ends of their lives. Their families took care of them, too. I wasn't a caregiver for them but I did visit them occasionally and help where I could. In addition to my own experience, I've spoken with many people who were or are caregivers for dementia and Alzheimer's patients.

My story is a cautionary tale. I'm trying to talk to each of you so you learn from my mistakes and be encouraged by our successes.

I hope my experiences will help you, whether you are a full-time caregiver or someone who occasionally interacts with an elderly loved one.

CHAPTER ONE

BECOMING A CAREGIVER

I have nothing to offer but blood, toil, tears and sweat.

-Sir Winston Churchill

YOU BECOME THE PARENT—and your parent becomes the child: that happens when you realize your parent's mental or physical ability is slipping to the point where your roles have begun to change. When this role reversal occurs, it is not the happiest time of your life, but it need not be the worst.

The first hurdle is deciding when that day has come. It may come suddenly with obvious signs of mental deterioration, or the realization that something is wrong may take a long time. Some people rush the day. The first "senior moment" or mistake is to some a sign that the elderly person is incapable of caring for herself. Sometimes it is done maliciously; the adult child who wants the parent out of his life or to obtain control of any assets. Some forgetfulness occurs at any time in life—the misplaced homework of a child; the misplaced key of a young adult. Then suddenly the misplaced item is evidence of aging. Not necessarily so, without a pattern of problems.

A personality change—a person who was very authoritarian becoming meek or a person who was very sweet and loving becoming belligerent—also can signal the beginning of severe problems.

The other side of this is not recognizing the day has come. You may be in denial because you don't want it to be true and don't want to face the future without a parent to lean on, however subtle or seldom the leaning may be. If you're not seeing your parents regularly, are you truly aware of what's happening? I knew a very concerned daughter who lived out of state. She spoke with her elderly parents often by phone and thought they sounded fine. They reassured her they WERE fine. When she finally came to visit them, she was stunned to find her normally tidy parents living in absolute squalor.

I certainly did not want to accept that my parents were beginning to have health issues. My father announced to my mother and me one day that he thought his hearing was deteriorating and he wanted to look into buying a hearing aid. My mother and I promptly said no, your hearing is fine. It wasn't fine, and he was right about needing a hearing aid. But I remember vividly how I denied he had any problem because, as I realize now, I didn't want him to have a problem or to admit he was aging.

As I've mentioned, I was born when my parents were about 40, so these issues arose earlier in my life than they might for others. It doesn't matter. When you recognize that your parents are aging, you must deal with the inevitability of becoming an orphan: the fact that you are 20, 30, 40, 50, 60, or older is completely irrelevant to your emotions. I consoled myself with the thought that I could drop dead myself at any moment and not have to face being an orphan. Not a very healthy consolation.

The fact that you are 20, 30, 40, 50, 60, or older is completely irrelevant to your emotions.

My mother had high blood pressure for many years. She started showing signs of senile dementia while I was in law school in the late 1970s. Mom became legally blind sometime after she became senile. This meant she could discern light and dark and some shapes. Dad had hearing loss, prostate cancer for which he had an operation, and heart disease. He had rheumatic fever when he was about 20 and apparently was left with an enlarged heart. He had two angioplasties unblocking the arteries around the heart. Both parents were found to be borderline diabetic. An EKG found heart damage to my mother's heart and she ultimately died of heart failure. Dad died of leukemia— 14 hours, HOURS, after being diagnosed with acute myelogenous leukemia.

My sister and her husband and daughter lived just two blocks from my parents' house. My sister did what she could to help, but her husband was a semi-invalid and took up most of her time. No other family could help.

Long Time Coming or Sudden

Sometimes, there is no mental deterioration as we normally think of it, but lapses in judgment. A friend of my parents was rather a tyrant in his own home. One day he was clearly ill, and his wife and grown daughters wanted to call for help. He ordered them not to call an ambulance; they obeyed—and to their horror—watched him die on the living room floor.

> # I went into the living room and found him sitting in a chair—and having chest pains.

My father was one of those without mental deterioration. However, one night I thought I heard him go into the living room. He often slept on the couch in there. I was about to roll over back to sleep, but I was nagged by the thought that he should be in bed. I went into the living room and found him sitting in a chair—and having chest pains. He knew he had a recently diagnosed heart problem and that he was probably having a heart attack. He didn't want to wake the household, though, so he just sat in a living room chair.

I got him into the car and to the hospital. He had had a very mild heart attack, caught in time, so the damage to his heart and his health was minimal. Afterwards I asked him to clarify his decision. He indicated he hadn't wanted to bother me.

"You didn't want to wake me and disturb my night's sleep?"

"That's right."

"So you thought you'd sit in the chair even though you knew you could die there?"

"Yes."

"So I would wake in the morning and find you dead, and you thought that was the best way to handle it?"

"Yes."

> # I slept very little, often only four hours out of 24, and very lightly, getting out of bed at any and every sound.

This bit of thoughtfulness on my father's part was, of course, ridiculous. But its effect on my life was profound. From that day until my father's death some 10 years later, I never had a full night's sleep. I slept very little, often only four hours out of 24, and very lightly, getting out of bed at any and every sound. Parents of infants will understand the lack of quality sleep I experienced.

* * *

The family had known for several years that something was "off" with Mom, and we attributed it to her growing older, although she was not yet 70. I personally consider that an early age to experience noticeable mental deterioration. I have read, though, that the first Alzheimer patient, a woman treated by Dr. Alois Alzheimer, was 51 when treated and 56 when she died. Alzheimer's can strike the middle aged as well as the elderly.

The turning point for my mother was one day when she was making dinner. She made somewhat elaborate dinners and this one consisted of a meat course, vegetables, potatoes for mashing, and gravy. All were cooking at the same time, and she was trying to plan it so everything finished at the same time. This can be a bit tricky for anyone. I heard her in the kitchen clearly upset.

When I went to her, she said something along the lines of, "I can't, I can't."

She could not decide what to do next.

I calmed her down and led her to the porch. We had a glider that she loved to sit on in the evenings, and I had her sit there. I went back and found that the dinner was almost finished. Everything was cooked and ready to be put in serving dishes except the potatoes, which needed mashing. From that day forward, she was unable to cope with anything the least bit complex, even though this had been something she did virtually every day.

> She was unable to cope with anything the least bit complex, even though this had been something she did virtually every day.

She had been a good cook, so I tried to have her help me with small parts of the cooking chore. We often made waffles from scratch so I asked her to separate the eggs so the whites could be beaten. Separating takes a certain knack but it was something she had done effortlessly for many years. This time she just stared at the eggs and was unable to act. Heartbreaking.

CHAPTER TWO

MY REALITY; YOUR REALITY

All happy families resemble one another; every unhappy family is unhappy in its own way.

-Leo, Count Tolstoy, *Anna Karenina*

Books for Caregivers[1]

I FELT AS IF I was in the middle of a battlefield with the enemy closing in on me and I grabbed the nearest weapon—a gun. I'd never handled one before, but: quick, I need to know how to fire it to save myself and my family. The only instructions in front of me are how to choose the right gun, its care and maintenance, and suggestions for target practice.

That's the way I felt about the books available to me for caregiving. Interesting information but not helpful for NOW. So much of the time, I was thrown into a crisis and I just wasn't prepared.

I read numerous books dealing with caregiving and caregivers. Unfortunately, I found they often ranged from misguided to insulting and on to impossible. Some were genuinely helpful, although even those could be overwhelming in scope and in the expectation of the abilities of a family caregiver.

I resented the authors who I felt described caring for the elderly as if they lived in what I call *The Donna Reed Show* utopia. If you believe that the typical household consists of a mother who provides gourmet meals made from scratch for her family for breakfast lunch, and dinner while dressed in a lovely gown, expensive pearls, and luxurious high-heeled shoes; handles all the chores from laundry to repainting the interior of the home without breaking a sweat; and without taking time away from her perfect family which includes children who get straight As and never get dirty—in other words a

1950s sitcom—then you can believe in what some of these experts say.

However, if you, like me, live in the real world, you will realize some experts do not portray real life, 24/7. Their theories sound great on paper, but I cannot believe some of these writers ever experienced anything remotely like what I faced in my 23 years as a caregiver.

YOUR reality might be as these experts describe, but if it is not, THAT'S OKAY! Mine was not, and I got through it and my parents did as well as possible. You can, too, and I hope with some input from me, my warnings, it can be less painful for you than it occasionally was for me. Each situation is unique.

As an example, dementia often is accompanied with anger, change of mood or change of personality. This occurred with my parents but not to the extreme that others experienced.

YOUR reality might be as experts describe, but if it is not, THAT'S OKAY!

Professionals suggest that caregivers not take anything the dementia patient says personally. That's true but very difficult to do. Intellectually I knew it wasn't personal, but my kneejerk reaction was to be more emotional than objective.

Your Situation

My cousin, who had to handle issues with both of her parents and now is dealing with her husband's dementia, pointed out to me that there is a very different dynamic at work when coping with a spouse than coping with a parent. I know she's right, but I cannot comment on caring for a spouse because I didn't have that issue. I can say the dynamics in my home were different when there were three of us than they were when my mother died and it was just Dad and me.

Another common suggestion is to have a friend stay for a couple of hours while you nap. This is great if you can get it to happen. I had an aunt who was willing to sleep in my mother's bedroom one night while Dad was in the hospital, and I slept for the first time in a couple of days. It's hard to find someone so caring, however. Your friend may be willing to come over but would probably like to spend the time chatting with you.

Keep in mind that you will probably lose friends during this period of being a caregiver—or more accurately, you will learn who your friends really are. Anyone who has not experienced the caregiver's life won't understand why you cannot get away to meet them, or if you do have a date set, why you might have to cancel.

You will learn who your friends really are.

Other suggestions for caregivers include keeping up hobbies and treating yourself well by buying new clothes, and so forth. Depending on your situation, you may be restricted in what you can do. My mother was very sensitive to my "noise" in the form of television and music. It made enjoying those things impossible— especially when she decided to watch TV with the sound extremely loud.

Taking care of oneself by buying a new outfit is also tricky when you have no place to wear it and your finances are suffering because you are working less or not at all in order to be the caregiver.

Professionals suggest you reconsider your approach to be certain you are handling everything as well as possible. As a practical matter, it is difficult to function at your peak when you never have a chance to step back and look at your situation objectively. When I was responsible 24/7 for 23 years, I was caught up in day-to-day living and had trouble being objective. As a family member, I didn't come into this difficult situation as an outsider, as does a physician, nurse, or physical therapist. This was my life; my parents were my support system, and the issues came up gradually.

Another suggestion is that if your siblings criticize how you care give, you ask them to take over for a day, or better yet, a week. If this is not possible because they live far away, they can volunteer for an organization dealing with dementia to see what people who have these problems are like. However, I suspect when volunteering like this, one is inclined to believe his or her parents wouldn't behave the way these patients do.

I realize it's very difficult to be part of the "sandwich generation" which cares for the younger generation as well as the older one. But it was also very difficult to take on the responsibility in my late twenties. Because I had to care for my parents for so long, I lost the chance to have my own family.

Some of the time that I was taking care of my parents, I did have an outside part-time job. It was difficult because, as I have mentioned, I often only slept four hours per night. I tried going to work on less than four hours sleep, but it just was not possible.

One morning after a poor night's sleep, I got ready for work as usual. I went to the garage and got into the car. I watched the garage door open...and the next thing I knew I was pulling into the parking lot near the public transportation that I took each day. I had driven the approximately three miles to that lot without being aware of it. That was terrifying. From that time on, I missed work whenever my parents' problems caused me to have less than four hours sleep. Ultimately, I had to give up working completely.

I cooked and cleaned, but I also cut hedges, washed the car, rotated tires, mowed grass, painted house trim, fixed the lawn mower, and repaired the dryer, because my parents didn't want to spend any money on repairs. Dad had always repaired everything, and if he couldn't, it fell to me. (I did auto body work too—really badly, but I did it!)

Creative and flexible!

Doctors often ask for an extensive evaluation of the patient including occupational therapy evaluation and neuropsycho testing. I couldn't get my mother to go to doctors much less submit to extensive testing. This wasn't a change in her personality—she never did go to a doctor if she could possibly avoid it.

You, as the caregiver, can cope with anything—just be creative and flexible!

13

CHAPTER THREE

THE CHALLENGES
PART ONE

I'm an old woman now, and nature is cruel.
'Tis her jest to make old age look like a fool.

> -From "Crabbit Old Woman," attributed to Phyllis McCormack[2]

A THUNDERSTORM USUALLY MEANT I could not leave the house. Mom would become terribly upset to think I was going outside. I found it nearly impossible to go to work when she was clinging to my arm, crying, and begging me to stay. I was only employed sporadically—part time jobs and temporary assignments. I never developed a good method to deal with this other than trying to ignore it. I think a caregiver has to prepare for this type of behavior—behavior that stems from fear. A good strategy probably would be distracting the person and slipping away while he or she is engaged in something else. I was not leaving (or trying to leave) my mother alone. My father was staying with her, so it wasn't a question of her being worried about being alone; she was afraid for me to go out into the storm.

* * *

> ## Just about everyone spoke too fast for her.

Mom watched television with the volume very high. When she blasted the TV, I don't believe it was because she was hard of hearing—that came later—but because she couldn't understand the people on TV who spoke too rapidly for her. She was trying to comprehend what people were saying and just couldn't grasp it. Just about everyone spoke too fast for her. One of her favorite programs was *Designing Women*, which ran from 1986-1993, but she had to stop watching it because the banter was so fast.

All television programs started to cause problems. Mom began to complain that there wasn't much to the shows anymore, and I finally realized that she turned them off when the first commercial came on, believing the program was over. No wonder they seemed so short; she only saw about ten minutes of them.

Mom was especially fond of a television show starring Tony Randall, which ran from 1981-1983, called *Dear Sheldon*. Actually, it was entitled *Love, Sidney*. Mom knew that the title of the show referred to the letters the main character had written. She "remembered" it as being how he BEGAN his letters rather than how he signed them. This sort of confusion—she insisted to everyone that the name of the program was *Dear Sheldon*—was one of the early signs of her dementia.

* * *

> # The symptoms of dementia and blindness were manifesting themselves simultaneously.

Mom's blindness went unnoticed by the family for a while. She had always been very nearsighted and the condition was so extreme that she never learned to drive a car. She faked us out, though, and we fell for it. For example, one evening at dinner Mom asked if someone would hand her the mashed potatoes. The bowl of potatoes was literally touching her plate. We pointed that out to her and she made some comment like, "Oh, silly me," and took the bowl and served herself.

We were oblivious to the fact that she could not see the bowl. The symptoms of dementia and blindness were manifesting themselves simultaneously, and sometimes we attributed an action or event to the wrong cause.

Mother had a horror of doctors. She had gone to a doctor for glasses when she was about 16 or 17 years old. She was working and could finally afford to go. The doctor prescribed glasses and she had that prescription filled. When she wore them to work the next day, she had more trouble reading than ever. Her supervisor pointed out that

15

glasses shouldn't be doing that to her. My mother went back to the doctor and found out that he had switched the prescription, so what he had written for the left eye was actually for the right. Mom had the lenses switched, but her skepticism about the medical profession deepened and she avoided doctors as much as she could.

* * *

Taking Mom to a wake caused her to become hysterical. She knew we were going to a wake when we got in the car but, of course, after an hour ride, all thoughts about the death of her nephew's mother-in-law were gone. When we got to the funeral parlor, relatives grabbed her and dragged her up front so she could pay her respects. Mother's eyesight was so poor she had no idea where she was; and then she suddenly realized she was looking down at a dead person. She started to scream in panic and hyperventilate. The well-meaning relatives had taken her when we first came in, and I didn't have a chance to intervene. I chased them down the aisle trying to regain control of the situation, but I was too late.

When her sister, Tish, died, Mom attended the wake and handled herself fairly well. She wasn't able to go to the funeral the next day, though; she was too upset. Oddly, she also thought she was now the only living sibling, completely forgetting her sister, Marie.

She had to have the purse in her lap at all times.

The Golden Girls Was Right—Not Letting Go of the Purse

A character on the television show *The Golden Girls*, Sophia, was always pictured with her purse. My mother didn't hold on to her purse in her own home, as did Sophia. However, when we went out she had to have the purse in her lap at all times. Places where she had normally been very comfortable, such as my sister's house two blocks from my parent's home, became challenging for her. She had to eat with the purse in her lap. This troubled and embarrassed my father greatly, and although he was normally a very quiet man, he yelled at her over this. My advice here is: do not fight this one. As ridiculous as it may seem to us, the challenged woman needs her purse. Let her have it. Ultimately, all the yelling, cajoling, reasoning, and tricking would not work. If she did set it down for a minute, she would suddenly panic and need it, NEED IT, again. I suspect this is always a losing battle. I would suggest that you pick your battles and let this type of thing go.

On a related note, my mother panicked away from home unless we were in the car. If we parked and then went in somewhere, she soon began fretting about the car. My father had a mild heart attack and was in the hospital. My mother noticed his absence. She was terrified that he might be dead. I assured her he was fine.

"If he's fine," she said, "then bring him home."

I had to take her to see Dad to prove he wasn't dead.

Well, I couldn't do that because he was in the hospital. Mom then thought he might not be dead but he was dying. I assured her he wasn't dying. Then you should bring him home, argued Mom. I told her that we couldn't for another day or two. Mother was fine with that explanation—for a few minutes. I went outside and soon Mom came running out of the house yelling that she couldn't find Dad. Again, I assured her he was in the hospital but fine. No, she insisted, he must be dead and I was keeping it from her. I had to take her to see Dad to prove he wasn't dead. She was reassured to see him at the hospital— for a few minutes.

Then she panicked that we could not get home because the car might not be okay where it was parked. She kept saying we had to leave and get to the car. I had no choice but to take her home, which calmed her but upset my father because he was ill and needed moral support for more than the brief time we were there. He also had trouble believing that she couldn't help herself with her panicking. Dad thought she was being terribly insensitive to his needs.

(When we got home, my mother noticed my father's absence and panicked that he might be dead. I assured her he was fine. If he's fine, she said, then bring him home. The cycle continued until my father was well enough to come home.)

Not Letting Go of the Chocolate Bunny

At Easter one year, I bought a six-inch chocolate bunny for Mom from Fannie May, a wonderful candy shop. It came in a white tray and I knew that Mom would be able to see the brown chocolate against the white, even though she was legally blind—as well as enjoy eating the chocolate. I brought it home and showed it to her. She held it in her hands and said she wanted some right away.

I said, "Give it to me and I'll take it to the kitchen and cut off some pieces."

> It was rather awkward cutting up a chocolate bunny being held in Mom's lap; but she was happy.

She said no and refused to give it up. She wanted me to bring the knife to the living room. I did bring the knife and it was rather awkward cutting up a chocolate bunny being held in Mom's lap; but she was happy. I believe she had been afraid that I would take the chocolate away and she wouldn't get it. AND she was clever enough to know that if she let it go she would have no way to get it back if I didn't bring it back. She couldn't see it, and she wasn't sure she could articulate it or even remember what it was she wanted.

Such treats became more and more important to Mom. We had a celebration for my parents' 65th anniversary at the house about one year before she passed away. She didn't seem really to grasp what was going on, but she did know we had a small wedding cake for dessert. Her whole focus that evening was on the cake and making sure she got to eat a slice of it.

Terrified of Respite Workers, Nurses, and Others

Conventional wisdom tells us that one cannot be a full time caregiver 24/7 without any breaks. The problem is, who can relieve the caregiver? My mother was terrified of any strangers in the house, so I could not hire a nurse or other caregiver. Mom would become very agitated when anyone other than my father and I were with her. Occasionally she was comfortable with certain family members, but they weren't available to stay very long.

The problem is, who can relieve the caregiver?

A recent trend is the opening of elder care centers that take seniors one or more days per week for several hours. The family can bring the person, or vans can pick them up and bring them home. This gives caregivers a break while professionals work with the elderly.

It would not have been an option for Mom, however, because of her fear of leaving the house and her fear of strangers.

Refusing to Leave the House

My mother got to the point where she absolutely refused to leave the house. I believe it was a self-preservation instinct. She knew she was having trouble coping with everything in her life, and at least in her own home she could feel safe. Even though my father and I would be with her, she could not be persuaded to leave.

Finally, we convinced her to ride in the car the two blocks to my sister's house. We got her into the car; we drove to my sister's house without my mother complaining or being upset. She would not, however, get out of the car. We had felt, my father and I, that we had won a real victory to get my mother out of the house, but we were wrong. She was feeling pretty comfortable in the car and wouldn't get out. We went back home. She was fine about getting out of the car and back into the house. Of course, she did not really KNOW it was her house. Being legally blind, she could not see it. Maybe she just trusted that we would not lie about where we were. We tried not to lie. We felt losing our future credibility was not worth it.

This refusal to leave the house meant that I could not take her to the doctor, podiatrist, or to the dentist. She couldn't have her hair cut. Fortunately, a friend of the family was a hairdresser and agreed to make house calls. This way Mom could have her hair trimmed and look and feel better. The doctor also was understanding and occasionally made house calls. Our house was only a few blocks away from his home. He sent geriatric nurses to check my mother. Mom accepted them as long as they were there only briefly and Dad and I stayed with her.

Inability to Discern Between Dream and Reality

> # I could not convince her that she had been asleep and not on the phone.

One day Mom awoke from a nap and informed my Dad and me that Dad's brother, Robert, wasn't selling his house after all. Actually, Robert was intending to sell his house and did so. However, my mother had a very vivid dream that Robert called, she answered the phone, and he told her he decided not to sell his house. I could not convince her that she had been asleep and not on the phone.

The Rose, Horse, Orange Test

A test was mentioned in the newspaper that was supposed to determine if one had Alzheimer's disease. The caregiver tells the person three unrelated words such as *rose, horse*, and *orange*, and explains that in a few minutes she will have to recite the three words back. I did it with my mother, telling her that it was a game and she should remember the words *rose, horse, orange*. I chatted with her for a moment and then asked Mother to tell me the three words.

> # "Rose, horse, orange?" Mom was indignant, "That doesn't even make sense!"

Mom asked, "What three words?"
I answered, "The three words I just told you."
"You didn't tell me three words."
"Yes, I did."
"Well, what were they?" Mother challenged.
"Remember? It was rose, horse, orange."
"Rose, horse, orange?" Mom was indignant, "That doesn't even make sense!"
Mom had no recollection of the discussion moments earlier that she was going to remember these three words, but she did know that they sounded very silly.

THE CHALLENGES
PART TWO

Which of you by being anxious can add one cubit to his span of life?

-Matthew 6:27 (Revised Standard Version)

Not Able to Peel an Orange.

I TRIED TO KEEP MOM busy by giving her little tasks around the kitchen. As I've mentioned, one of the earliest signs of her dementia was when we were making waffles from scratch and was unnerved by the idea of having to separate egg whites from yolks. Another day I gave her an orange to peel. She said she was sorry, but her mother always did those kinds of things and she didn't know how to peel an orange. I should mention that Mom was from a very poor family, the youngest of seven children who had been abandoned by their father. My mother had an orange once a year as a Christmas present, so she did not grow up knowing how to peel oranges.

It was almost as if she was back to a time when she was about six years old. Some days she would wake up and ask for her mother. The first time upset me quite a bit. Even though I was maybe 40 years old at the time, when my mother seemed afraid and asked for her mother, it just threw me.

I learned to say, "She's not here right now; can I get you something?"

After just a few minutes, she would come back to the present and realize her mother wasn't around anymore. One time Mom woke up and asked for her father. When speaking to me, she had always called Dad "your father." When she asked for her father, I asked her if she meant Paul Schoen. I never heard Mom or any of her siblings refer to their father other than by his full name, "Paul Schoen." He had not been a part of her life after she was about four years old, so I didn't really think she meant him. She said no not him but couldn't think of the name of person she wanted. I realized she was trying to say "your father" rather than "my father." I brought Dad to her and she was fine.

Another time, Mom seemed to be about 16 years old. At first, she was disoriented, and I had to explain to her that Dad was her husband, George Tarnow. She said she was too young to be married. I assured her she was married to him.

Mom clearly remembered dating him but not marrying him and kept repeating, "I married George? I married George?"

She was okay with it, just surprised. As I wrote in the preface, they married when Mom was 20 and Dad was 23; they had dated for several years before that, so she was very clear about who he was.

Another time Mom seemed to be about 16 years old.

A third time she seemed to be about 36. Mom remembered having one child, my sister, but could not remember that she had a second child. Mom insisted she had only one child, and, since I'm 12 years younger than my sister, for 12 years, Mom DID have only one child.

Mom actually seemed to be reliving parts of her past.

Turning on the Water

Generally, I felt confident that Mom was safe if she was in another room. It seemed okay to leave her alone because she seldom did unusual or dangerous things. One day, though, Mom turned on the kitchen faucet and left the room. The drain was closed, but I don't know if Mom closed it; sometimes the water pressure caused the stopper to go into place. By the time I came into the kitchen, we had a small flood. The water leaked a little into the basement, too.

One day, though, Mom turned on the kitchen faucet and left the room.

This presented a new dilemma. If she could do that, she could do any number of other things that could damage the house or worse, hurt her. However, this was just one incident. Did that justify round the clock surveillance so that she was never alone in the room? Could she be allowed in the bathroom by herself? Since it was just one occurrence, I decided to keep monitoring Mom but not get additional help unless we had another "incident." As it turned out, we didn't have any more problems.

Paralyzed Not Knowing Which Faucet Handle Was for Hot Water

One heart-breaking incident occurred when my mother wanted to rinse her hands under the kitchen faucet. She stood paralyzed in front of the sink. I asked her what she needed. She wanted to use cold water because she was afraid she might burn herself if she used hot, but she could not remember which was the cold and which was the hot handle. Mom could not bring herself to just turn one on and test it. I waited with her for a few minutes, but she could not make a decision, and eventually I had to turn it on for her. I cannot guess how long she would have stood there confused and afraid.

Turning on the Stove

Mother also turned on the burners on the stove. This was very early in her illness. She had done some laundry and hung it out to dry, and then realized it was starting to rain. She ran inside to get my help. I had been making dinner and had a saucepan on each of the four burners. I turned off each one as I walked past to the back door. Mom followed closely behind me, and I knew she was checking each knob to be certain it was in the off position—at least that was what I thought. She had the lifetime habit of double-checking the knobs anytime she passed the stove.

> # When checking the burners to be certain they were off, Mother actually turned them on.

We quickly took the wash off the line and had it inside before it started to rain heavily. I went over to the stove, and all the burners were on, and they were on high. When checking the burners to be certain they were off, Mom actually turned them on. Fortunately, no damage was done. The food wasn't even burned, as we had not been outside for more than a few minutes. Here again, I had to make a decision. Mom was functioning at a fairly high level. Yet, she was losing her common sense, and was already well on her way to being legally blind. Should she be closely supervised every moment? This has to be a judgment call on the part of the caregiver. I never did do anything to keep her from the stove, and that was the only incident Mom ever had with it.

Answering the Phone.

> # Other times Mom said pretty ridiculous things on the phone.

I had an issue that probably would not come up today. We had a stationary landline telephone and no simple way to hide it. Today, of course, we have portable phones for our landlines and, also, cell phones. Mother ran to answer the phone every time it rang. It wasn't easy to wrestle it out of her hand. Sometimes she spoke sensibly enough but when she hung up, she didn't know who it had been on the other end. Other times Mom said pretty ridiculous things on the phone, and I was never sure to whom she said them. I can't imagine how many messages were lost. At the time, I was actively looking for work and was expecting calls to schedule interviews.

Friends and family did not realize that Mom was having the problems that she was. Oh, I told them, but she sounded so darn sensible for much of the time that it was hard for them to believe me. People don't want to acknowledge that someone close to them is slipping away.

One day the three of us, Mom, Dad, and I went shopping for a Super 8 movie camera—a precursor to video cameras. We came home and the phone rang. Mom answered the phone; it was my sister. To our amazement, Mom told her we had bought her, my sister, the camera for as a gift. Dad and I were trying to stop her from talking with no success. When she got off the phone, we asked her why she said that. Her explanation was that my sister had asked what was new, and she couldn't lie and not tell her that we had bought her a camera for Christmas.

Of course, it's not lying to keep a Christmas gift a secret, and we had bought it for ourselves; it wasn't a gift. Dad and I didn't know how to handle the situation. Give my sister the camera for Christmas?

Buy a second one for her? Explain the situation? It's much more difficult to explain to people than you may imagine. In this case, Dad and I explained to my sister, and she understood because she was beginning to realize Mom's limitations.

At first, I was in denial.

In these early stages, we didn't know really what was happening to Mom. The doctors weren't sure at first either. Initially, I was in denial. When I did know what was happening, I told friends and relatives that didn't believe me. They either didn't understand the extent of the problem or were in denial themselves. As I write this, Mother's decline seems so clear. At the time, however, I was just feeling my way through a fog of issues that I couldn't understand and I couldn't fully articulate.

Bathing

Another early sign of Mom's dementia was her refusal to bathe. In her defense, she had extremely dry skin and even with the doctor recommended lotions, she was uncomfortable after a bath. When my father and I tried to get her to bathe, her usual answer was that she just had just recently taken a shower, but, of course, that wasn't true.

When I tried to make her bathe, she had what they call a catastrophic reaction. That's when a person has a very strong reaction to a minor event. Mom wouldn't bathe if I just talked to her about it. But she would become hysterical, cry, yell, and become red in the face if I tried to steer her toward the bathroom.

Birthdays

Mom had no sense of the passage of time.

I told Mom that her only granddaughter would be turning 20 years old soon. The day before the birthday I reminded her again and Mom said, "Oh yes, she's turning 21."

I explained that she would be 20.

Mom replied, "But I'm sure last time, you said she was turning 20 so this time it should be 21."

Yes, "last time" I did say 20, but that wasn't a year ago; it was two weeks ago. Great that she remembered our conversation and her granddaughter's age; unfortunate that Mom had no idea how long ago that conversation had taken place. Mom had no sense of the passage of time and often confused recent events as having happened long ago. She also thought some things that she had done the year before had only recently happened.

CHAPTER FOUR

SOME THINGS THAT WORKED
PART ONE

Do not go gentle into that good night.
Rage, rage against the dying of the light.

-Dylan Thomas

AS A CAREGIVER, you want to do all you can to keep the elderly person as engaged in life as possible. However, when you want to involve people with dementia or failing faculties in any type of activity, you cannot approach them head on. If you directly introduce the project, it seems as if you are issuing a challenge; it seems like a test. The person will often become agitated and unable or unwilling to cooperate. Again, be creative and flexible in approaching the elderly with activities.

Jumble Game

> She would get very upset that she was doing so poorly even though she was doing very well.

Before her mental decline, Mom was great at playing the Jumble game that appeared in the newspaper. It's an anagram game with five- or six-letter words. She could solve all of the words instantly and certainly without writing anything down. When Mom became blind, I found that I could read the letters aloud to her and she would come up with the correct word almost immediately. In fact, Dad decided he would play, too, and he wrote the letters down as I said them. He would just be writing down the last letter when she would shout out the answer. Occasionally, however, she would not be able to get one of the words. This created a new problem. Mom thought she was missing most, if not all, of them when, in fact, she was answering most of them. She would get very upset that she was doing so poorly even though she was doing very well.

I had to stop the game about a year before she died. Her hearing started to decline and she couldn't distinguish between many of the letters that rhyme: B, C, D, E, G, T, etc.

Probe Letters

We played Jumble another way, too. In the 1970s a game called Probe came out which consisted of among other things, a deck of cards, each with a different two-inch tall letter on it. I would pull out the five or six letters from the Probe deck that made up the Jumble word. Then I would put these letters into an envelope. I left those envelopes lying around.

As I've said, I couldn't come straight out and ask her to try the game because that upset her. This way, she would find the envelope on her own, look at the letters, and try to make words. I had to do many things in such an indirect manner. Not only was it was too much pressure to ask her to look at letters to see if she could make a word; it was even too much pressure for her to be handed the envelope. If she found the envelope on the kitchen table, she could take the letters out and make words, and enjoy the process. Today, of course, we can make our own large letters on a computer.

Christmas Lights

Although Mom was born very nearsighted, she became legally blind only after she was senile. She was not able to learn any coping strategies for her blindness. I tried to brighten her life as much as possible. Fortunately, she could tell the difference between light and dark. I bought colored Christmas lights and put them in the living room for her to enjoy. I also was able to find lights that played Christmas songs and blinked to the beat of the music. Since they provided sound as well as light, she took great pleasure in them.

Music

Mom enjoyed all kinds of music, so when she became legally blind I provided more music for her. She was not able to turn on a radio or tape player herself.

> She delighted in lyrics such as, "potatoes are cheaper, tomatoes are cheaper, now's the time to fall in love,"

The songs that she really enjoyed were old novelty songs that all seemed to have lyrics relating to food. She often sang them while she was cooking when I was a little girl. She delighted in lyrics such as, "potatoes are cheaper, tomatoes are cheaper, now's the time to fall in love," "yes, we have no bananas, we have no bananas today," and "you're the cream in my coffee, you're the salt in my stew."

We had a lot of fun singing them even though neither of us could remember all the words or sing on key. Of course, we sang them mostly in the kitchen.

She had enjoyed an old television program called *Sing Along with Mitch*, which featured the Mitch Miller Orchestra. I was able to find an audio tape and play her old favorites of that.

Providing the music that the senior enjoyed in years past not only gives pleasure but also engages the person. Music may trigger memories, and reminiscing is a positive activity as well.

Photos

Showing the elderly old photographs and letting them reminisce is an excellent tool. Again, it has to be done with no pressure if there is any slowing of mental ability. If you show the senior a photo and ask who it is, it can cause that person to be upset. Typically, they cannot remember the person's name immediately and become annoyed with themselves for not remembering. This can escalate from annoyance to great agitation. However, if you allow them just to look at pictures, the memories usually will surface on their own and the person will fill comfortable talking about them. So many of the activities have to be approached obliquely so that it is something the senior comes to naturally and spontaneously, rather than something that is being forced and feels like a test of one's memory.

> # So many of the activities have to be approached obliquely.

If the person is blind, you can encourage general reminiscing by relating bits of old stories; then the memories and stories may come to mind. If you say, "Tell me about Uncle Ambrose," the person may very well shut down. Worse, the person may become flustered, worried, sad, or other negative feelings may arise from being unable to do something he or she feels should be so simple. A better approach for Mom was for me to say, "Wasn't there a time when you were at the beach...?" Telling the beginning of a story that I had heard her tell before was also very useful.

Painful Knees

Dad went through a period of being grouchy, but I realized the arthritis in his knees was bad. Dad never liked to take anything for pain if he could help it. We were in the living room and he was watching the game show, *Wheel of Fortune*. Dad was deaf so he didn't watch much television, but he could follow this show without the sound. I pulled up a stool next to his chair and rubbed his knees. He appreciated it because it not only felt good at the time, his knees hurt a little less for the rest of the day.

It became a daily habit—I rubbed his knees for a half hour every evening.

Dad was very grateful and kept asking, "Why are you so good to me?"

I never told him, but I also was being good to ME. He was in a much better mood all day, every day, as a result of these massages. I was doing it so I didn't have to be around such a grouchy person!

SOME THINGS THAT WORKED
PART TWO

Most folks are about as happy as they make up their minds to be.

-Abraham Lincoln

Set the Table; Knives, Forks, Spoons, Plates, Cups, Glasses

I WAS UNDER the impression that since Mom was having so much trouble remembering and understanding, she would not know how to set the kitchen table for a meal. To make it easier—what I thought would be easier—I told her to bring out knives, forks, spoons, plates, cups, and glasses.

She tried to follow along with what I was saying and said, "Knives, glasses...."

Then she said that she had to go to the bathroom. She stayed in the bathroom for almost a half hour. I think it was because she couldn't remember that list of items I had rattled off unthinkingly to her, and she was upset. Or she didn't want me to know she couldn't follow my directions. In any case, she didn't come out of the bathroom until dinner was on the table. I tried variations of explaining the things to bring out to set the table. But nothing I said was clear to her.

Finally, one day I asked, "Could you set the table?"

And she did.

Mom could remember the words, "set the table," much more easily than, "bring out knives, forks, spoons, plates, cups, glasses." More importantly, she knew what "set the table" meant and she had no trouble doing it. I thought I was doing a good thing by explaining everything that had to be done because I was so sure, from the way she handled other things, that she no longer knew what "set the table" meant. I recommend phrasing things in various ways until you find what is most easily understood.

> # Mom could remember the words, "set the table," much more easily than, "bring out knives, forks, spoons, plates, cups, glasses."

Also, written lists can be very helpful. I couldn't use anything written because of my mother being legally blind. (Actually, she could read very large black letters and distinguish a short word. However, she could not read a sentence because after reading two or three words, she would forget what the first word was and lose the train of thought.) I was limited in having to give direction orally; hopefully you will have other options. Written lists were very helpful for Dad.

Washing Dishes

> # She washed each dish carefully, rinsed it under the faucet, and placed it in the drainer.

Another very effective way of having Mom do things was just to get her started. I wanted her to try washing dishes. I filled the kitchen sink with warm water and dishwashing liquid and had a few plates in the sink. I asked Mom if she would do the dishes. As usual, she said she couldn't. I got her to go to the sink, though, and I gently took her hand and put it in the water.

Mom exclaimed, "Oh!" and reached for the dishrag.

She washed each dish carefully, rinsed it under the faucet, and placed it in the drainer. As I previously mentioned, she had been afraid of turning on the faucet because she could not remember which was the hot or cold handle. Now she was using the faucet easily. Next, Mom reached over to the counter to feel for more plates. When she finished the plates, cups, glasses, and flatware, she walked over to the kitchen table and felt around to see if there were more dishes to be brought over to the sink and washed. This occurred about two weeks before her death.

It was interesting to me that about a week later she had some type of brain scan in the hospital. The results didn't come back until the day she passed away. The doctor said that Mom should have been a complete vegetable because her brain was highly calcified. I wish that doctor could have seen Mom skillfully washing those dishes!

Having had success with this technique of gently leading Mom to the dishes in the warm dishwater, I tried it again the next day. It happened to be Mom and Dad's 66th wedding anniversary. When she finished the dishes, I explained to her that it was her anniversary, and she should go to Dad and say, "Happy anniversary."

She pointed out that she got her sleeve wet. I said that was okay and she should go tell him "happy anniversary" now. I led her over to where my father was sitting and said that Mom had something to tell him. Only a few seconds had passed between my coaching her and her talking to Dad. However, her memory was incredibly short. I told her to go ahead and tell him.

She hesitated and then blurted out, "My sleeve got wet!"

Oh well, I tried. The lesson for me was this: Mom's memory was very, very short; less than a minute. Yet, the "reminder" in the form of a wet sleeve enabled her to remember that part of our little conversation. Perhaps if I had given her some other "prop"—I can't think of what that might be for someone with limited vision—the prop could have reminded her of what she was going to say. When I told her to tell Dad "happy anniversary," she WANTED to do it. I wasn't forcing her—but she couldn't remember. She could not forget, though, that her sleeve was wet because it was a constant reminder until it dried.

Changing Clothes

Mom did not change clothes. She wore her nightgown and robe virtually all the time. Yes, cleanliness was an ongoing battle. Changing made her uncomfortable and I, with my dad and sister, did what we could to get her to change her clothes. She physically could handle dressing and undressing; she didn't want to do it.

Mom did not change clothes.

When changing her clothes took the three of us, because she fought it. Mom screamed and cried, too. It took so long...well, let's just say we didn't have her change every day.

Cabinets

When Mom was just beginning to show signs of dementia, I decided to make things as easy as possible. Our dishes were not arranged in the cabinet very well. The cups, glasses, and small lunch plates were on the bottom shelf. The dinner dishes, which were a bit heavy, were on the second shelf. Mom, Dad, and I were all short people and it was a stretch to reach the second shelf, especially to lift out something heavy. I decided to put the heavy dishes on the bottom shelf and the lunch dishes on the second shelf to make it easier. It was easier—for a few hours. My mother then complained that she couldn't find the dishes. Her eyesight was quite poor at that point, but Dad and I didn't know it. I put the dishes back the way they were.

Socks

Mother could discern light and dark, so I had her pair up socks and roll them into balls. She liked being busy with tasks like this. She could often tell which socks matched, not because of color but because of the size, shape, and stitching of the socks, which she could feel. (I found it interesting that she tried to match a bright red sock with a brilliant blue one: she explained that those two colors appeared the same to her). I put the socks that I knew she couldn't identify in pairs and let her roll them up and put them in the laundry basket.

> I found it interesting that she tried to match a bright red sock with a brilliant blue one…those two colors appeared the same to her.

Deafness

My father became increasingly deaf with age. He couldn't hear the television unless it was blasting. We found a simple solution. I bought a radio that had the TV band on it, too. He put that next to his chair and tuned it to the same station he was watching. He had an earphone so he could turn up the volume as much as necessary to hear the program without bothering Mom and me.

CHAPTER FIVE

SPECIAL FRUSTRATIONS

What doesn't kill us makes us stronger.

-Friedrich Wilhelm Nietzsche

THE ABOVE QUOTATION was one of my mother's favorite sayings. She especially enjoyed reciting it to me whenever I was complaining about a new challenge.

I always retorted with, "Yes, but what if this does kill me?"

I never got an answer.

If Nietzsche was correct, I should be pretty darn strong by now. In addition to the day-to-day frustrations, there were certain events that were especially difficult for me.

Mom and Dad swore I was crazy one day when I got a mosquito bite. I came in the house to get an anti-itch medicine we always used. It was a liquid in a cylinder that looked like a brown fountain pen. I was having trouble finding it, and they both asked what I was looking for and I explained. They said they never heard of such a thing and were certain we never had it. Not only did we have it, but they really liked the product and told others about it. I kept searching. They asked again, and I described it as almost looking like a cigar—a brown cylinder.

"Okay," said Mom, "You think we have a special cigar that makes bites stop itching?"

And that's when they both explained to me in no uncertain terms, over and over, that I was "insane." I got in my car, drove to the drugstore, bought the product, brought it home, and showed it to them. Their response?

"Oh."

They didn't elaborate. I don't know if either of them then remembered seeing it before (and I did eventually find our original cylinder to show them, too) or if it was all new to them, but we never discussed it again. It's terribly frustrating to be in a situation where you are caregiving alone, feeling isolated, and you have two people "gang up" on you in this way.

"Is it possible that I AM losing my mind?" I wondered.

I had no one to talk to, no sounding board, no reality check. This event was the sort of frustration that makes one feel very alone.

"Is it possible that I AM losing my mind?" I wondered.

* * *

I cooked every day, trying to make the meals as healthy as possible. Mom and Dad were on low-salt, low-fat, and sometimes low-sugar diets.

I was grateful we had a television in the kitchen because having it on while I worked for hours preparing meals relieved the tedium. Then one day Mom wandered in the kitchen while a commercial was on the set. The advertising included classical music playing in the background. Mom demanded to know the title of the music and the composer. I didn't know. Mom declared that if I did not know what I was listening to on the TV, I was not "allowed" to have it on. She turned it off. I couldn't reason with her, so I kept if off for some time. I sorely missed have the TV for company during the hours I spent cooking, but it was better than agitating Mom.

* * *

I was having trouble reaching some cook pots that were in the back of the bottom shelf of a cabinet under the kitchen counter. I sat on the floor to pull them out. Dad found me there and wanted to know what I was doing. I explained. He said I should either squat down, which I had tried, but it was too tough on my knees, or simply bend over. I stayed as I was, on the floor dragging out the pots I needed.

Dad walked over to the phone and called my sister explaining to her, "Georgette has lost her mind."

To Dad, sitting on the kitchen floor, even briefly, was bizarre. Even though he disliked using the phone, he was so distraught that he felt he needed outside help. Daily chores became very difficult when incidents like these occurred, as they did occasionally.

The rarity of these incidents with both Mom and Dad seemed to make them worse when they did occur. Much of the time, they were behaving normally and I was lulled into thinking they were doing pretty well. When they did something odd, it was a shock. I think if they did strange things every day, I would have been more prepared.

* * *

When I started law school, Mom told me I should come home each day and teach her exactly what I had learned. That way, she said, she would be a lawyer, too. Of course, that was impossible. After I became a lawyer, Mom bought a book about how to avoid lawyers by writing your own will. She proceeded to lend it to anyone and everyone who showed the slightest interest. Apparently, she intercepted some of my phone calls, and friends and family members who were contacting me about making wills never got to talk to me, but did get that book.

> ## After I became a lawyer, Mom bought a book about how to avoid lawyers.

Mom was clearly acting inappropriately because of the senile dementia. It still hurt, though, not to have the support and respect of Mom and Dad. Since I dedicated myself to their care and cut myself off from the outside world, I never did have support. I was wrong to keep myself from the help I truly needed.

* * *

> ## I actually broke a chair once purely out of frustration

Sometimes I wished my sister would help me. She lived a five-minute walk away from us, but she was caring for her husband who was a semi-invalid. Unfortunately, when I called her house (remember, this was before cell phones) her husband would answer and hang up on me. Not so much being rude, I suspect, as just having a short attention span.

The conversations would go something like me saying, "Hi, how are you feeling?" and he would say, "Not too good," and hang up.

I always assumed my sister realized I called and didn't care. Now I know she was not aware that I called; I just wished she would call and check on our parents more often, but she had to handle her own caregiving.

I actually broke a chair once purely out of frustration. I was having a particularly bad day dealing with Mom and I was in the dining room. I picked up one of the wooden dining room chairs and lifted it about a foot off the floor and slammed it back down. A leg broke off. In my defense, I still think it should not have broken so easily. I told my aunt about it and she drove over, took the chair, had it mended, and brought it back. She said we need not tell anyone about the incident. I am telling about it now because I believe everyone needs to realize how very difficult, sad, and FRUSTRATING caregiving can be.

* * *

Mom, being nearsighted, wore glasses all her life. One day she just stopped wearing her glasses. After a few days, I insisted she try them on again. She put them on, but said that they made her dizzy. Finally, we were able to get her to the eye doctor. He asked Mom if she could read the chart on the wall.

Mother asked, in all seriousness, "Where's the wall?"

Mother asked, in all seriousness, "Where's the wall?"

She could see a little but when the doctor finished his examination of her eyes, he explained to us that she was legally blind due to macular degeneration. Glasses couldn't help her anymore.

* * *

I wasn't able to have privacy in the bathroom. I didn't lock the bathroom door because encountering locked doors seemed to upset Mom. It's not very relaxing to take a bath and have someone become

38

hysterical outside the door. But when I left the door unlocked, she generally walked in. Sometimes she would use the toilet while I was in the bathtub. A hot bath was not a refuge any longer.

I even had to cut short my visits to the bathroom as Mother seemed to have problems and call for my help every time I went!

* * *

When I was in law school in the late 1970s, it was clear that many law firms were not hiring women attorneys, or just hiring a few. I wanted to open my own law firm. I confided this to Mother, and she said go ahead and do it. I pointed out I needed some money to rent an office—maybe as much as $25,000 to get me through the first year or two. Not a problem she said, she and Dad would be glad to lend it to me. I knew that they had very substantial savings, so they could lend me the money without any hardship. When I graduated and said I was ready to do it, Mom had no recollection of our discussion, and said that she and Dad certainly could not afford it. It never occurred to me that she didn't mention it to Dad or that she was losing touch with reality. I was too embarrassed to ask Dad or to put him on the spot. I started job hunting.

* * *

Everyday chores were frustrating, too. Because both parents were on low-fat and low-salt diets, my twice weekly grocery-shopping trips each took three hours or more. How could I find things that were healthy that they would enjoy? Even if I were making homemade meals, I had to make sure of my ingredients.

> # My twice weekly grocery-shopping trips each took three hours or more.

For example, we used to eat spaghetti with a store-bought spaghetti sauce in the jar. I couldn't find low-salt spaghetti sauce, so I had to make a sauce using tomato sauce—when I could find a low-salt version. A better alternative was for me to make the sauce from fresh tomatoes from the grocery store. The best option would be to make sauce from my own homegrown tomatoes from the yard. So we went from having a simple meal of spaghetti with jar sauce to me feeling so guilty that I tried to grow large quantities of tomatoes just to make into sauce!

Sometimes we had meals that had salt in them, even though we tried to be careful of salt intake. I reluctantly served my father a bowl of soup from a can—a flavor he especially enjoyed. The doctor wasn't being terribly strict at this time, so I knew having salt occasionally probably wouldn't hurt him. I watched in dismay, however, as Dad went to the cabinet for salt, and added it to the already salty soup.

* * *

Mother liked to talk. A lot. She went through a period where she chattered on, not quite making sense, for more than an hour at a time. During one such episode, I left Mom, talking to herself, and joined Dad in the living room.

"I had to get away," I told Dad, "I couldn't listen to her voice anymore."

"Someday you're going to miss that voice," counseled Dad.

He was right, of course, but at the time it was difficult to be patient.

Dad was allowed to have crispy fried chicken IF he removed the skin first. I had made a point of restricting my diet along with my parents' diets so we all ate the same food. One evening we were having chicken and I dutifully removed the skin and left it on my plate. Even though he knew better, Dad ate his chicken with the skin on. Then he asked if I intended to eat the skin from chicken. When I said no, he picked it up off my plate and ate that, too!

> ## Dad was allowed to have crispy fried chicken IF he removed the skin first.

I bought a salt-free soup as a base for a dish I was planning for dinner. Mom and Dad found the soup and made it for lunch without me knowing it. They hated it and threw it out. I discovered what they had done and had to start over with planning that day's dinner. The next time I went to the store, I had to buy the salt-free soup again to make the recipe I originally intended to make. When my parents saw it, they complained that they didn't like that soup. It took a lot of explaining that it was just one ingredient of many in the recipe.

CHAPTER SIX

PARANOIA

Paranoia strikes deep, into your life it may creep.

-Buffalo Springfield, from the song, "For What It's Worth"

PARANOIA WAS ONE of the most upsetting symptoms of my mother's dementia. She became very suspicious and distrustful, and this was one of the very first symptoms she displayed.

When she was still in her sixties, she bought two packages of lotion. Each package contained a bottle of lotion and a free small tube of hand cream. One package was for her, the other for me. Mom thought it was a great deal and a nice little gift. That was thoughtful of her, but it was not the kind of lotion I used. I stored mine on the floor of my closet, not knowing what else to do with it. Some weeks later, I came home from work, and as soon as I entered the house, Mom started screaming at me, calling me a thief. She had bought lotion for herself, she said, and when she went to use it, she couldn't find it. She had searched my room and found it on the floor of my closet. Mom had proof of my theft!

I knew where she kept her toiletries, so I calmly went into her bedroom, looked around, and found her package. I explained that she had purchased two and given me one, but I didn't want it and to take it back.

How awful that Mom could think I would take something of hers (and especially galling since I didn't like the lotion). I didn't realize it was just the start of a long road of dementia. These paranoid outbursts were probably the most personally upsetting of all the symptoms.

Next, Mom began insisting that I bought her Christmas, birthday, and Mother's Day gifts only because I chose items I wanted, and then I wished her dead so I could have them. She repeated this to me every time I gave her a gift. I stopped the presents because her

42

accusations were as upsetting to her as they were to me. Not a healthy situation. Then family members realized I wasn't giving her presents on special occasions and I was criticized for that. I explained the problem, but no one seemed to believe me. Clearly a no-win situation.

> # Mom began insisting that I bought her…gifts only because I chose items I wanted, and then wished her dead so I could have them.

* * *

Mother had been a fresh air fiend, having the windows and doors open early in spring through late fall. One evening, Dad was in bed asleep and Mom woke up and wandered into the living room where I was watching television. She became very upset that the front door was not shut; only the screen door was shut and locked. I explained that it was fine because I was sitting right there, and I would shut and lock the door in a half hour. I wanted to watch a rerun of *M*A*S*H*. She wouldn't accept that and stood by the screen door, without moving, for the full 30 minutes until the TV program was over. I was trying to show her that everything was all right and we were safe. I also didn't want to cave into any more of her demands that were fostered by her growing paranoia. I don't think either one of us "won" that night. I know I didn't have the relaxing evening I hoped for.

> # She came running out screaming that I had laid a trap to murder her.

One day, early in the course of the dementia, Mom went into the bathroom to take a shower. She came running out screaming that I had laid a trap to murder her. I had been in the bathroom immediately before she went in and left my razor on the side of the bathtub. The tiny disposable plastic razor with its cap securely fastened over the small blade couldn't hurt her, but to my mother it was proof of my homicidal intent.

Before Mom became senile, she pulled some of her old high-heeled pumps out of her closet. Instead of discarding them, though, she put them in a carton in the attic. A few years later, she was up in the attic and found the box. She confronted me with a pair of shoes in her hand. Mom was very angry and told me that I was a terrible person. When we had gone shopping, she said, I had begged her to buy me those shoes, and then I not only never wore them but also hid them in the attic. Of course, I never asked Mom to buy me shoes, and these were her quite worn old shoes, but I had to bear the brunt of her distrust once again.

* * *

As I mentioned earlier, from time to time, Mother would wake up from a nap and announce news that she had just heard. They were only her dreams and the stories were usually harmless. Some of the dreams, however, were more sinister. Our neighbors of about 20 years had built a brick barbeque in their backyard. When Mom awoke, she was convinced that these lovely people were disposing of bodies in the barbeque. The story evolved, and she soon believed that they were killing babies and disposing of them in that barbeque.

* * *

In the last year of her life, Mom became too afraid to go down into our basement. She believed people regularly came in from outside. The last time she was in the basement, which had a beautiful party room, was her 65th wedding anniversary. Mother's only grandchild's bridal shower was down there, the following year, but Mom was too afraid to come downstairs with us.

In the last year of her life, Mother became too afraid to go down into our basement.

---

* * *

Being a caregiver was so tedious and boring, I looked forward to doing volunteer work. Our American Legion Auxiliary unit had an annual card party and raffle to raise operating funds for the year. I had been a bookkeeper and I was also a lawyer, so the officers asked me to handle the simple accounting needed for the raffles. I did it once and I enjoyed it. I need something to do outside the home. The women of the unit were happy with my work and invited me back the next year. However, the next year, they did not offer me the job. That hit me hard because I had so few outside interests and nothing to give me a sense of satisfaction and self-worth. Years later, after Mom had passed away, I was talking with some of those officers and I found out why they didn't want my help. They explained that they wanted me to volunteer, but my mother forbade it. She said that there might be a money shortage and she didn't want me to be held responsible. Only a few hundred dollars were involved and I was an attorney, but Mom was too afraid to let me handle it.

When I felt I could get away briefly once or twice a month, I contacted the bar association to volunteer in my neighborhood. The only slot available was to help the seniors at a home with their legal problems. I declined to the total mystification of the volunteer coordinator. She thought it was a perfect fit with my background. I couldn't handle dealing with any more elderly people—I just couldn't.

* * *

One day I left Mom alone for a few minutes. In that time, the minister of our church called at our house. Mom liked him, but when he came to the door, she wasn't sure who he was. The dementia was getting worse than I realized. She refused to let him in because of her intense fear of strangers. He seemed a little miffed afterward, but I was so grateful that Mother had such great instincts for self-preservation.

> When mother fell asleep on the living room couch, she would lie very still. I couldn't tell if she was breathing.

* * *

Mother wasn't the only one to have irrational fears; I did, too. It became increasingly difficult for me to give Dad a hug because I could hear his heart beating, and each beat seemed like it might be the last.

45

After his heart attack, I couldn't get the idea out of my mind that his heart might stop just as I hugged him.

When Mom fell asleep on the living room couch, she would lie very still. I couldn't tell if she was breathing. I often went up to her, afraid she was dead, and hoping she wasn't, to check her breathing. As a caregiver, you need to find ways to not stress yourself out the way I did; clearly, I handled this part of caregiving very poorly.

"Oh, if we had known she was YOUR mother we would have taken better care of her!"

Sometimes I had good reason for paranoia—or at least worry. Our neighbor, a former nurse, visited her mother in the hospital and found the nurse on duty was an acquaintance of hers. When the neighbor explained who she was there to visit, the nurse exclaimed, "Oh, if we had known she was YOUR mother we would have taken better care of her!" It's rather chilling to think that some professionals provide different levels of care.

* * *

My mother's personality change was extreme. She had been wonderfully creative. The following is an excerpt of one of the many stories she invented for me.

Pink Curls…a Christmas Story

Santa had his nose buried in a large black book in which he kept a record of all of the toys he had made during the year. As she watched him, he looked up from the book and Mrs. Santa saw the frown on his face.

"Are you still worrying about Janie's doll?" she asked.

Santa just stared straight ahead as if he didn't hear her.

Mrs. Santa thought about the first time she had heard about Janie wanting a doll with pink curls. Alex brought Janie's letter in the first mail delivery after Thanksgiving. Alex was the pilot of the airplane that brought mail and supplies to Santa at the North Pole. With the letter, Janie enclosed a page torn out of a coloring book and on it was a picture of a beautiful ballerina doll.

The doll was colored pink from the top of her head to the tip of her toes. She had long pink curls, the color of strawberry ice cream, and on her head rested a tiny crown set with pink pearls.

Janie had never asked Santa for any presents before. She was so sure Santa would bring her the doll that she had already picked out a name. She was going to name her "Tina."

It was more than three weeks since Santa received Janie's letter and he still did not have pink hair for her doll. Santa and his helpers had tried every kind of dye but they could not make the pink color that Janie wanted. Santa was worried that Janie would be sad if the doll wasn't just like the picture.

CHAPTER SEVEN

HUMOR

And laughter oft is but an art
To drown the outcry of the heart.

-Hartley Coleridge (son of Samuel Coleridge)

SURPRISINGLY, TAKING CARE of the elderly and particularly someone with dementia is not without its humorous moments. At first it seems wrong somehow to laugh, but my sister, niece, and I actually sat down and discussed the issue. We realized that dementia is never funny, but if a particular incident was funny, we just had to laugh. The days were rather grim anyway, and there would be no actual harm in laughing. Sometimes it was gallows humor; sometimes you laugh so you don't cry; and other times I was laughing at myself.

Gelatin was a popular side dish at our house. I would cut up some fruit and put it in the gelatin, and this fruit salad would be good for two or three days. Occasionally, I added yogurt. One time I decided to use a yogurt that had strawberries at the bottom. The yogurt itself appeared to be white. I added it to the gelatin, which happened to be green and lime flavored.

The result was a very tasty GRAY gelatin. In case you're wondering, gray is about as unappetizing a color as you can imagine. I had put other fruit in it, too, and it tasted very good. Really. It just looked awful. Usually, Mom, Dad, and I finished the gelatin in two sittings. This gelatin just kept reappearing at the table. Dad couldn't stand more than a spoonful at a time, and Mom's eyesight was still good enough to let her know how awful it really looked. If they had simply shut their eyes when they ate it, they would have been fine.

* * *

From time to time, Mom would lock me in the basement inadvertently, thus making herself secure—and me stuck. This was before cell phones. One time when this happened, my folks couldn't hear me banging on the door. I could have gone outside, around to the front, and rung the doorbell, IF I wasn't in my pajamas and slippers, and if it hadn't been snowing outside.

> I cannot tell you how much time I spent during those years banging on the ceiling with the broom handle.

Fortunately, we had an extension phone in the basement, so I called my sister and explained the situation. She then hung up with me and called the house. My parents answered the phone; she told them I was in the basement. The door was unlocked. I was lucky; sometimes they didn't hear the phone. Occasionally, hitting the basement ceiling with a broom, right under the room they were in, brought results. I cannot tell you how much time I spent during those years banging on the ceiling with the broom handle.

Other times, a basement can be useful to a caregiver. Recently a friend mentioned that she, a single woman, and her widowed mom bought a house together when the mother was first starting to show some slight signs of dementia. While living in the house, the mother was diagnosed with Alzheimer's. This friend said she specifically selected that house because it had a finished basement so she knew she would have a refuge to go to if she had to get away from her mom for a little while. Going to the bedroom or bathroom doesn't help. Locked doors tend to upset dementia patients—and they usually go into any room with an unlocked door.

* * *

Once, Mother experienced confusion with our tablespoons and teaspoons. She was drying the dishes and when she came to the spoons, she said she didn't know which was a tablespoon. I showed her the tablespoon, then picked up a teaspoon indicating it was a teaspoon.

Mom replied, "You don't have to tell me about teaspoons because I'm ALWAYS able to pick THEM out." If you have only two kinds of spoons, teaspoons and tablespoons, and you always know which are the teaspoons, how can you not know which are the tablespoons?

These goofy little everyday occurrences can be frustrating, but they also can be funny.

Mom was watching TV and came to find me to say she could not work the remote and so she wasn't able to turn off the TV. When I checked the TV, it was off and I thought she was really, really out of it. The same thing happened the next night with Mom trying to turn off the TV after the nightly news. Finally, I realized the TV was on a sleep timer and it turned itself off AFTER she left the room to find me. For a few days, though, I thought she was completely loony thinking there was a television program on the dark and silent set.

* * *

One day when they were just beginning to decline, Mom and Dad went shopping. Mom's sight was very poor, by this time, as was Dad's hearing. I stood at the open front door watching them as they left the house and walked to the garage.

"George, I hear a cardinal!" exclaimed Mom, "can you see where it is?"

Dad frantically looked in all directions, not knowing where to turn because he couldn't hear it.

"It sounds like it's over there!" reported Mom, waving her arm wildly.

Between them, they tried to find the cardinal and I quietly closed the door. It was a funny, sad, poignant moment and I didn't want to intrude as they worked as the team they always had been to discover the elusive bird.

* * *

She generally sang in the bathroom.

Mother went to the bathroom—sometimes out of necessity but sometimes, I think, just to hide out when life became too challenging for her. She generally sang in the bathroom. Not in the shower, but while using the potty. Almost always, the song was the "Star-Spangled Banner." You are supposed to stand whenever there is a live performance of our national anthem, so Dad and I, and any visitors used to debate whether we should be standing while Mom sang her heart out in the john.

* * *

One lovely lady who suffered from senile dementia was taken out to dinner by her family including her daughter, Mary. The next day a neighbor asked how the restaurant was. Mary knew her mother had no recollection of the event and watched as she covered in a very charming manner.

She simply said, "Oh, I'll let Mary tell you about that."

> It is quite common for dementia patients to be able to fool and charm people...for a long time.

The mother very cleverly avoided answering and prevented further questions; it is quite common for dementia patients to be able to fool and charm people who are not close to them, for a long time.

I knew one woman who was 99 and suffering from senile dementia. She was eating the liver sausage sandwich that had been prepared for her. I knew what it was, but to make conversation I asked her what she was eating for lunch. She replied that she wasn't sure, but she thought it was some kind of fish and that it was very good. I'm guessing that her sense of taste was failing her, but she enjoyed her food anyway.

* * *

I had to be careful to balance the desire to be light hearted with preserving my mother's dignity. Once when I was trying to make her hurry up, I said, "Come on, quick like a bunny."

Mom stopped and glared at me.

"Quick like a bunny?" she asked stiffly.

I realized it was something I said to children, and even though Mom was very childlike, she still had enough pride to be offended at my comment.

I tried to treat my mother with respect at all times but as playfully as possible. I used to tell her, "If you want to eat, you have to work."

Of course, I would feed her and feed her well no matter what, but I wanted her to feel like a contributing member of the family. Therefore, I didn't hesitate to tease her a little, or play little tricks. We always wanted to have fun in the past, and I wanted to continue that. So, on one occasion when we were having cake with frosting, I cut a slice for Mom and then said to her, "Doesn't this smell good?"

She took the bait and smelled the cake slice on the plate I held in front of her. And yes, I did, ever so slightly, push the cake up to her nose. The very tip of her nose got frosting on it. She thought it was funny. More importantly, she felt like we were not walking on eggshells around her. We treated her as normally as possible.

> # One time Mom walked past me in her robe and she "rustled" very loudly.

Mom especially loved desserts, and cookies became her favorite. She seemed to have a sort of survival instinct and she would take a napkin and surreptitiously pocket extra cookies whenever she could. I would notice her pocket bulging with cookies. One time Mom walked past me in her robe and she "rustled" very loudly. I couldn't imagine why. A quick check of her pockets gave me the answer. She had found some of my individually wrapped cough drops and put a fistful in her robe. I made her turn them over to me because they were not candy, they were medicated, and she wasn't supposed to have them.

We went to a baby shower at my cousin's house. I was chatting with people and not watching Mom closely. I suddenly realized she was taking cookies from the tray and wrapping them in napkins and putting them in a pocket. I led her away from the buffet and seated her by the table. My cousin asked what was happening. Embarrassed, I explained that she took cookies whenever she could. He knew about her dementia. Without another word, he stood up, went to the buffet to retrieve the cookie tray, and placed it in front of Mom.

"Take all you want," he told her kindly.

He handled the situation so well—Mom was happy with the cookies and I stopped feeling embarrassed. Secretly, I was proud of my mother that she had the instincts to hoard food in an attempt, I think, to care for herself as well as she could.

* * *

At home, Mom could easily walk past a person without seeing them because of her poor eyesight. Other times she spoke to floor lamps thinking they were people. One day, as I was standing in the kitchen, she asked me where the toddler came from. I couldn't figure out what she was talking about.

> Mother could easily walk past a person without seeing them because of her poor eyesight.

"What toddler?" I asked, totally mystified.

"Over there," she gestured impatiently.

I looked around wildly trying to imagine what she could mean. Finally, I realized that she was looking at a 24-can case of Coca-Cola in its distinctive red and white packaging. Standing on end it appeared to be a small child to Mom.

Another time I was standing in the dining room, and she passed me going from the living room to the bathroom. She ignored me because she couldn't see me. As she passed I stretched out my arm as if I were a tollgate.

"Where do you think you're going?" I asked playfully.

"To the bathroom."

"Well, if you want to pass me, you'll have to give me a nickel."

Mom made an elaborate show of turning her pockets inside out.

"I don't have any money," she reported, clearly understanding that we were teasing.

"Well," I said, "I'll settle for a hug."

This was a bigger deal than it might seem. Mom was never one to hug us very much. In extreme cases, when I was very upset, I would get a hug. These hugs were very brief and ended with Mom saying, "That's enough now."

> # Mom grabbed me and started humming as she danced me across the dining room floor.

This time, Mom grabbed me and started humming as she danced me across the dining room floor. It was a beautiful moment, totally unexpected. She was, by the way, a wonderful dancer while I charitably can be described as having two left feet. At this point in her dementia, she didn't know who I was other than I was someone always in the house. After a quick spin around the room, she went to the bathroom.

* * *

Five months before Mom's death, her only grandchild got married. I was trying to keep Mom as a functioning part of the family as much as possible. I asked what she thought would be a good wedding shower gift. She was somewhat upset at the question. Questions are difficult for dementia patients. They can talk about things randomly, but questions generally put too much pressure on them. Mom said she didn't have any ideas. I pressed her a little.

Finally, she said that blankets were always nice. I followed her suggestion as best I could when I selected something from the bride's wish list: Mom's gift to her granddaughter was a king size down quilt.

Mother's dementia combined with the blindness made her oblivious to her surroundings most of the time. I managed to have Mom and Dad attend the wedding and reception even though I was in the wedding party because a neighbor, a nurse, agreed to come with us and care for Mom.

We got to the church with no problem. Mom and Dad were in the second pew and I was in front with the wedding party. During the service, the bride and groom went to their parents and grandparents. The bride went to my mom, her grandmother, and greeted her.

Mom recognized her granddaughter even if she was hazy on where she was, and said, "Whatcha doing, honey?"

The bride didn't miss a beat, "I'm getting married, Grandma."

This story has already reached legendary status in our extended family.

> # "Whatcha doing, Honey?"
> # "I'm getting married, Grandma."

Some humor came out of extreme frustration. When I was unable to get Mom to bathe for several weeks, I finally called my sister to have her help Dad and me get her showered. I actually blurted out, "Please come over and help me hose down the old lady."

I never called my mother an "old lady" before, but I was so aggravated with my inability to handle what seemed like a simple task that I said it that way.

* * *

My friend, author Tom Wolferman (www.tomwolferman.com), writes about his caregiving from a comic perspective. In the following excerpt from *Prairie Dogs Are Contagious*, one of a series of caregiving essays, he described the realization that his mother was falling victim to dementia:

Finally it was the growing clutter of notes and paperwork that flagged her decline. Once meticulously maintained, her house slowly was becoming disheveled. So was her head.

She had started documenting minutiae about baking cookies. On October 29, 2001 she made three batches of "Marge Riemer's Oatmeal Cookies" on an insulated pan in the lowest rack of 335-degree oven. On November 16 she baked 46 oatmeal cookies from Marge Riemer's recipe for a total of 20 minutes. On December 10, she produced three more pans of Marge Riemer's oatmeal cookies at a baking time of 14 minutes each.

Throughout the house we would find the recipe for Marge Riemer's oatmeal cookies. No one in the family ever recalls meeting Marge Riemer. If my mother wasn't slipping into dementia, clearly she was involved in some sort of black market cookie cartel.

* * *

Dad liked to inject a little humor in his day, too. If I were unwise enough to say something like, "As long as you're over by the counter, please give me the bread," I soon would have a loaf of bread flying at me. Bags of potato chips sailed across the kitchen, too. I think silly little things like that kept us sane.

When we went grocery shopping, the same thing happened. Dad would select a loaf of bread and toss it to me as I stood by the cart. In retrospect, I'm surprised we were never thrown out of the store with his habit of tossing unbreakables around.

CHAPTER EIGHT

THE UNEXPECTED

Great necessities call out great virtues.

-Abigail Adams

Giving Medicine

GIVING MY FATHER his medication was not a problem. He never wanted to take any medicine unless he absolutely needed it, so he seldom took anything for a headache. Nonetheless, he was always very careful to follow his doctors' directions completely, so he always took the medicines they prescribed. My mother, on the other hand, posed problems for me when it came time to give her her pills. Because of the dementia, I had to hide all medication from her. I don't think she would ever have taken medication on her own, but I couldn't be sure. As I mentioned, she found some cough drops that she thought were candy.

When it was time for her medication, I often spent about a half hour to get her to take her pills. First, I had to bring out the bottle of pills. Then I had to bring the tablet to her with a glass of water. The water would be too cold. I would have to get another glass of water, which invariably was too warm. Usually the third glass would be okay. Then she would argue that she didn't have to take any medicine. Next, she would need to know what it was for. When I finally convinced her she needed to take it, she would start to put it into her mouth. At that point, she would often say she really shouldn't because, she would explain, she only took what her doctor had prescribed for her. I would convince her that this was what the doctor prescribed for her. She, again, would begin to take the pill but then stop to ask the name of the doctor who prescribed the medicine. We would go around and around like that for a while, and finally she would take the pill. Exhausting and frustrating.

> # We would go around and around like that for a while and finally she would take the pill.

Once I was running late for an appointment. I didn't have time to give Mom her medication. I called my sister who lived nearby and asked if she could give Mom the pill. My sister came right over. She took the bottle of pills from me and handed them to Mom. My sister was finished—that was her idea of giving Mother her medicine.

First, I explained, you cannot let her have the whole bottle of pills because who knows how many she might take. Secondly, Mom was unable to get a glass or water for herself. I had a frustrating time teaching my sister how to give my mother her medicine. It wasn't rocket science—give Mom a pill and water and make sure she takes the pill—but there was an art to getting her to actually take it. What my sister was thinking? If I called her to come over because I didn't have time to give Mom her medicine, why would she think it was a five-second process of handing over a bottle of pills? Yikes! My sister did have her own cross to bear with a husband who was a semi-invalid.

When you have to give medication, I hope you have someone like my father to give it to. However, be prepared; you may have a more challenging person in your care. Go with the flow, and figure out the easiest and safest way to get the job done. Creative and flexible all the way.

> # The hospital staff kept talking to him in the ear with no hearing aid figuring that was the "good" ear. He never even knew they were talking to him.

Interestingly, when my father was in the hospital during one of several of his stays, I was told he absolutely refused to take his medication. I couldn't believe it and when the nurse offered the medicine when I was there, he took it very willingly. He told me, and I believe him, that no one tried to give him the medicine before that. What could have happened was he didn't SEE the medicine and didn't hear the request. Dad had a hearing aid in one ear; the other ear was completely deaf and could not benefit from a hearing aid. The hospital staff kept talking to him in the ear with no hearing aid figuring that was the "good" ear. He never even knew they were talking to him.

Lucid Moments

> In the week before Mom died, my niece, who was in her twenties, called her. My niece told her she was her granddaughter, and for the first time in years, my mom knew who she was and chatted with her.

My mother had a few lucid moments in the last years of her life. One was, well, horrible. Mom suddenly became aware of her situation and she said, "Something terrible is happening to me."

She seemed to know her mind just wasn't working right and she didn't know what to do about it. She was extremely agitated. The moment passed quickly and she settled down to her calm, but oblivious, self. I would have loved to have her back to being lucid but that wasn't possible. And I wouldn't wish that terror she experienced during those few minutes on anyone.

In the week before Mom died, my niece, who was in her twenties, called her. My niece told her she was her granddaughter, and for the first time in years, my mom knew who she was and chatted with her. That's a memory my niece will cherish forever. I cannot explain why it happened, but it just did. The whole experience of living with someone with dementia has many incomprehensible moments.

Two other times Mom became lucid momentarily. One time I came home from a bad day at work. I did work sporadically. I went into my room and, assuming she couldn't hear me, I cried. She burst into my room, AND knew who I was, AND asked me what was wrong. I started to explain, and she hugged me a let me cry on her shoulder. She started to tell me that these things happen and aren't worth crying over, but before she could finish the sentence, the dementia took over and she started rambling on incoherently.

The other incident was very similar with her comforting me when I cried. Apparently, when baby cubs are in distress, the momma tiger outranks the dementia patient and the tigress comes to the rescue. I cannot explain what happened, but hearing my crying just jerked her out of her fog, if only for a few minutes. After days, weeks, months, and even years of the same thing day after day, suddenly there can be a surprise like this that is as inexplicable as it is unexpected.

I was astounded; she not only was correct, she was fast in her calculations.

Mother was never completely in the fog. I had an opportunity to go shopping for clothes one day, and when I came home, I was telling Mom and Dad what great bargains I got. I said something like, "This was regularly $40 but I got twenty-five percent off."

Mom promptly said, "Oh, you paid $30."

This from someone who was having so much trouble with day-to-day living. I was astounded; she not only was correct, she was fast in her calculations.

Any strength a person has when healthy seems to be the strongest trait in the dementia patient. An accountant or bookkeeper will probably be good at arithmetic up to the end of his or her life. Mom was not a bookkeeper, but she was better than average with math. She was an excellent speller and that is why she was able to work anagram type puzzles in her head until she was too deaf to hear the letters read to her.

When Mom first began having symptoms of dementia, she could still do her normal chores around the house. She did laundry by gathering the clothes from the hampers, putting them in a laundry basket, and then taking the washcloths and towels from the bathroom and adding them to the basket. Before she actually took the dirty laundry downstairs, she would stop to put up fresh towels. One day she did that, took the load downstairs, and began doing laundry.

Then, as I watched her, she came back upstairs saw the towels and took them down believing they were dirty and she simply had forgotten them. She put clean ones up. I stopped her as she began to do the whole thing again—believing the new fresh towels to be dirty. She had no problem doing the laundry, but she no longer could remember what she had just done.

CHAPTER NINE

THE HEALTH CARE INDUSTRY
PART ONE

What do you see, nurse...what do you see?
Look closer...see me!

-From "Crabbit Old Woman," attributed to Phyllis McCormack[2]

Dealing with More Than One Issue at a Time
Mental Decline and Legal Blindness

ONE THING HAS ALWAYS annoyed me about the medical profession. Normally I have the greatest respect for nurses, physicians, technicians, and medical writers—everyone in the health care field. But there seems to be this notion that you can only have one thing wrong with you at a time. I am somewhat allergic to the chlorine in pools. I don't go in them because I get severe sore throats. I also was diagnosed with osteoarthritis in both knees when I was 24. I went to the doctor one day, and she said I should exercise more. She recommended jogging. I pointed out that was impossible because of the arthritic flare up I was experiencing. She then said I should swim. I mentioned my allergy. She said I had to choose one of the two. Apparently, in her world, one can be allergic to chlorine or have arthritic knees but not both.

This phenomenon was especially difficult with my mother. I was told one of the best ways to work with a senile person was to show them old photographs. It IS a wonderful way to get them remembering about the past and talking about it, but it can't work with a person who is legally blind.

Georgette H. Tarnow

Doctors Who Are Critical of You

You may have read that you are in a partnership with the medical personnel. You, as the caregiver, work hand-in-hand with the physicians. Ideally, this is true and we did have a general practitioner who usually treated me as a partner. However, it is very difficult to find physicians who will "partner" with you. Some doctors tend to be quite critical of caregivers even when they are following the doctor's orders.

The doctor began shouting at me.

One physician told me salt was very bad for Dad and I had to eliminate it from his diet. I did extensive research on sodium in the diet. At the next checkup, the doctor asked if I had followed his instructions. I indicated I had and that Dad was on a "low-salt diet." The doctor began shouting at me that it was to be a salt-free diet, NOT a low-salt diet. I pointed out that on planet earth, one cannot consume only salt-free things. FRESH fruits and vegetables have naturally occurring salt in them. Our water has sodium as well. Finally, he calmed down. This doctor was close to our family and I couldn't have anticipated his reaction. He was one of the best at making me a partner.

Apparently I should have know what the doctor MEANT and not what he WROTE.

Another physician told me to follow the prescription he gave me for Dad exactly. He specifically wrote that the generic medicine was fine. The pharmacist recommended the generic to me. When I brought Dad in for his next checkup, he was not doing as well as the doctor had hoped. I showed him the medicine and he went through the roof. Why, he asked, did I get the generic drug? I answered that he specifically wrote on the prescription that it could be filled with the generic form of the drug. He finally had to admit that was true but still blamed me for getting the generic drug. Apparently I should have known what the doctor MEANT and not what he WROTE.

None of my father's drugs were covered by insurance and they cost hundreds of dollars each month. Certainly we would buy the more expensive name-brand drug over the generic if it was needed, but where it wasn't we tried to be frugal because of the large amounts of money involved.

Just finding a doctor can be a tricky business. My father had a terrific cardiologist who was out of town when my father had a mild heart attack. By some fluke, no one was covering for him, so I took Dad to the emergency room. He was assigned a general practitioner, and soon, a cardiologist. The latter doctor did not have the best reputation and I didn't like the way he handled Dad. My sister and I wanted her husband's cardiologist who had a good reputation and was a genuinely nice guy. I called him, but he didn't want to take Dad on as a patient because on paper it looked like he would be the fourth physician in a day to take the case. It showed we left the first cardiologist (who was on vacation), and then left another doctor (the GP), and finally that we were leaving the cardiologist assigned to him (whom we DID want to leave). He felt we must be awfully difficult people if we kept changing doctors. Even with his personal relationship with my sister, it took a lot of talking to explain we liked the first cardiologist but couldn't reach him, and the others were just assigned to us on an emergency basis. He finally took Dad as a patient and, I believe, ultimately prolonged my Dad's life. To add to the confusion, that first cardiologist whom we liked and this last one who turned out to be so good for Dad had been professional partners but recently separated. Even though we lived in Chicago, it seemed like the world of medicine was pretty small.

Fighting for the Patient's Dignity

Don't let anyone treat them without respect, as if they are not quite human.

Whether your parent or other loved one is merely elderly, has heath issues, or is suffering from dementia, part of your job will be to fight the medical establishment and others for his or her dignity. Don't let anyone treat them without respect, as if they are not quite human. You may have to battle to make people understand that they are dealing with a human being.

At one point, I had hospital nurses treating my father very well. I commented on it and one nurse said, "When you care, we care. When we see how important a person is to the family it makes us care that much more."

I can believe that. A woman in the room across the hall from my father's hospital room yelled a lot. The staff ignored her. One day her yelling seemed more pitiful than usual, and I peeked in her room and saw her on the floor. I immediately summoned the nurses. They ordinarily would not have ignored a patient who shouted, but she never stopped yelling. No one ever visited her either. Well, that's not quite true; one day, a group of family members stomped into her room, stayed a few minutes and left, never, so far as I know to return.

> I pointed out we were slow in realizing it could be a heart attack because Dad did not sit in a rocking chair but was chopping roots for two full days.

My father had his first, mild heart attack when he was 84. He had the classic symptom of an aching left arm. However, this was on a Monday and he had spent Saturday and Sunday with an ax chopping the tree roots out of the lawn. He got tired of using his right hand so he chopped with his left arm, too. He thought the achiness in his left arm (often a symptom of heart attack) was the result of all that unaccustomed work. We went to the doctor who sent him to the hospital, and the tests showed he was having a heart attack. The doctors in the hospital said he was old and that could be the end. I pointed out we were slow in realizing it could be a heart attack because Dad did not sit in a rocking chair but was chopping roots for two full days. He also was very active in a number of organizations, serving as secretary for one and treasurer for another. This sort of stereotyping of the elderly, assuming they are not active, must be fought.

Dad was in the hospital one January, early in the month. The nurses seemed to think of him, not disrespectfully, but as if he were "out of it." I then heard them talking about New Year's Eve, and how they had just rested, and not gone out to celebrate. I chimed in and told them about the family party Dad attended to welcome the New Year. It was perfectly true and they began to look at him with a new respect, that he was a fully functioning person who happened to be elderly and ill.

Mom's Monitor

> # The medical personnel told me that my mother's skin should not be so dry, it could lead to problems—making it clear it was my fault.

About a week before my mother died, she was in the ER. Something was wrong with her—she became faint while in the bathroom. At the ER she seemed fine, though. The doctors decided to have her wear a Holter monitor for 24 hours to monitor her heart activity. The parts that affix to the chest—the electrodes—wouldn't stick to Mom because her skin was so dry. They had to put long strips of tape to hold it in place.

The medical personnel told me that my mother's skin should not be so dry, it could lead to problems—making it clear it was my fault. It was a very nasty situation with me feeling I was a bad daughter who let her parents down. Mom often wouldn't let me touch her. I had the lotion that our family doctor recommended for her and I applied it as much as she would let me, and I encouraged her to use the lotion, too. Because Mom had high blood pressure, I couldn't force her to do anything. If I tried, she would become upset and red faced. I had been warned by her physician NOT to excite her.

When Mom was in her twenties, strangers would come up to her on the street and ask her what her secret was for her gorgeous skin. She had an incredibly lovely complexion. The "secret" was that, even as a child, she had extremely dry skin. As a teenager, she never once had any sort of breakout; on the downside, her skin aged rather early in life.

> # We each held one of her hands and didn't let go for hours until she became sleepy and we put her to bed.

They sent Mother home with the Holter in place: it couldn't be touched for 24 hours. Dad and I got her into her nightgown and she kept "discovering" the Holter on her chest—it was a box about the size of a pack of cigarettes but heavier—and telling either Dad or me that she found this thing. She wanted to pull on it, so we had her sit on the sofa in the living room, and we turned on the TV. Dad sat on one side of her and I sat on the other. We each held one of her hands and didn't let go for hours until she became sleepy and we put her to bed. She didn't like it and wanted to pull away, but we needed the information the Holter was gathering for the doctors to be able to help her. It was quite an ordeal.

We went to the hospital the next day and found the Holter had come detached. They checked how many hours it actually recorded. It hadn't recorded at all! The connections must have fallen off her chest as soon as they were attached, and we had that long, miserable night for nothing. Mom died within a week, of heart failure.

When Dad was in the hospital after a mild heart attack, I received a phone call one evening from the hospital nurse indicating that Dad had some sort of attack. My sister and I couldn't reach the doctor but shortly thereafter ran into him at the neighborhood homeowners meeting.

We asked the doctor how Dad was doing. He said he's doing fine. I said even though such and such happened? He didn't know what I was talking about and immediately contacted the hospital. As it turned out, Dad had had a problem but the hospital did NOT notify the physician. He was furious, of course, and made sure that the staff never made that mistake again.

An answering service refused to forward my call to the cardiologist even though my father was having chest pains. The woman at the service said she didn't believe it sounded serious, and she could choose not to contact the doctor, at her discretion. I took Dad to the ER and the situation was handled. Later I explained to the cardiologist why he wasn't notified. The next time we went to see him, he made a point of saying he had changed answering services.

THE HEALTH CARE INDUSTRY
PART TWO

I was sick and you cared for me.

-Matthew 25:36 (New Living Translation)

DAD WAS HAVING CHEST PAINS and since he had ongoing heart issues, I took him to the emergency room. It was about 6 AM. Right before the chest pains started, he had eaten most of a box of chocolate cookies—the kind with the chocolate frosting. The heart problem was easily resolved. However, the blood test showed his sugar levels were high. The emergency room doctor decided Dad must have diabetes. His reasoning was that it was a very high reading on a test when my father "must" have been fasting for many hours. The doctor assumed Dad had been asleep prior to having chest pains. If he had shared this with me, I could have explained that instead of sleeping and fasting, Dad had been awake and had a huge intake of sugar. Dad was put on a non-insulin diabetes medication. The medication did not seem to agree with Dad. I spoke with the doctors and learned that if he missed a dose of this particular medicine it would not hurt him. That is not true of many medications, but in this case, it would be all right. However, if he took too much of this medication, it could lead to complications.

> I brought him orange juice—not only would he not drink it; he was angry that I would offer him orange juice that made him queasy to look at.

Within a few days of starting this new medication, Dad was exhibiting the signs I was warned to watch for. I decided to withhold one dose. Still, it seemed as if Dad's side effects were getting worse and included nausea. I was supposed to give him orange juice when these symptoms occurred. Dad was rather deaf and didn't have his hearing aid in his ear. I brought him orange juice—not only would he not drink it, he was angry that I would offer him orange juice that made him queasy to look at when he was already feeling so nauseous. I couldn't make him understand that he HAD to take it to counteract the effects of the medication because he couldn't hear me and he was too ill to understand.

We went to the emergency room again. Our family doctor couldn't make it right away, but the physician who was substituting for him had been apprised of the situation. He wondered if it was a flu, or one of many other possibilities. I asked him about the medicine for diabetes because it was a new medication for Dad, and because I believed Dad was having the side effects I was told to watch for. The physician explained that the medication must be working because his blood sugar was rather low. I said that I had withheld the most recent dosage and told him the exact time that I had given Dad his last dose. If Dad had been diabetic, the doctor said, his blood sugar would have been quite high after missing that dose This proved to the doctor that my dad never did have diabetes and that his symptoms were, as I thought, side effects from a medication he should never have been given.

My dad recovered very quickly, and the physician was happy that I could explain in detail what had happened. Otherwise, it would be a long process of elimination as to what may have caused Dad's symptoms.

Later I questioned the family doctor about Dad's original diabetes diagnosis. He said he had thought that Dad had a mild case of diabetes, and if he DIDN'T take medication for it, the problem would become acute some YEARS later. Dad was already 90. The doctor further explained that if the dosage of this particular drug was more than Dad needed, it could lead to death within one HOUR.

> Here I knew that missing a dose would not endanger Dad and I decided to withhold his medication. That may have saved his life.

Often a missed dose can be life threatening. Here I knew that missing a dose would not endanger Dad and I decided to withhold his medication. That may have saved his life. To best serve those in our care we have to learn a lot about medications. It takes a bit of work AND physicians who are willing to work with you, the caregiver.

In this situation, my father, who was normally quite sharp, was oblivious as to what was going on. He knew they thought he had diabetes but was not up to speed as to the type of medication he was given and its side effects. He fought me on the orange juice because he could not understand what was happening.

I always made a point of getting medications refilled when my parents still had several days' worth of their drugs left. One time I couldn't get to the pharmacy because of an emergency and went for the refill at the last minute. The pharmacy was in the middle of changing over their computer system and couldn't find the prescription in their database, so they refused to refill it. At that point, wouldn't you know it, I couldn't get in touch with the doctor. We only had a few hours because it was an important heart medication that Dad would soon need. Caregivers need to plan ahead—who would have thought that I would have an emergency AND the pharmacy would lose our records at the same time? I believe it's best to have a general practitioner who knows what is going on with the specialists, and who works with them. I was able to contact our GP sometimes when I couldn't reach a specialist. He could prescribe the refill or know if a certain side effect was dangerous, and so forth. Get as many medical people on your side as you can; those who will work with you to ensure their patients get the best care possible, even in the middle of the night.

During one of Dad's checkups, the nurse wanted to review his diet. She wasn't sure he was eating healthy enough, although we had reduced his intake of fats and salt. I finally became so exasperated that I asked her if she was afraid that Dad, who was 89, would die young. She had to admit that whatever he had been eating, it served him very well, and she had no further suggestions. When Dad was born in 1907, his life expectancy was 46 years. His mother died in her early 50s and his father in his early 60s. By this time, Dad was quite surprised that he was still alive!

I finally became so exasperated that I asked her if she was afraid that Dad, who was 89, would die young.

Please learn all you can about every medication or treatment given to the person in your care. The caregiver needs to know what the medication does and any possible side effects to watch for, as well as knowing about refills and if generic substitutions are okay. Also, ask what if one dose is accidentally missed or late, what if several doses are missed, and what could happen in case of an overdose. The caregiver needs to know this information to be aware how serious an incorrect dosage may be. An overdose can happen, especially if the patient has access to the medication.

> # The caregiver needs to know what the medication does and any possible side effects to watch for.

I also suggest caregivers learn how to help a person who is choking or who needs CPR, and also how to help someone who has fallen. Ask your physician or nurse to help you with these. We were very fortunate to have a retired nurse living next door. She was quite close to my parents, and was a wonderful help and source of information.

When I had to take either parent to the emergency room, I could list his or her ailments, their medications including dosage, and how recently the last dose was given. I could also explain anything that might have precipitated the problem. On several occasions, I gave my explanation to a nurse, and when the ER doctor came in he said, "I understand you're a medical professional." Our family physician encouraged me to keep learning.

Fooling or Charming the Doctor

> # The doctor promptly asked mother who the president was. She responded with a disgusted, "Oh, him!"

I previously mentioned that dementia patients can often fool people outside their immediate circle into thinking they are fine. They often use charm to avoid questions they cannot answer. This charm can also be used on health care professionals. I explained to our family physician that Mom was having definite problems; that she probably had dementia and was clueless about the world around her. The doctor promptly asked Mom who the president was.

She responded with a disgusted, "Oh, him!"

I am certain she had no idea who the president was.

However, the doctor didn't like the policies of that particular president and he proceeded to launch into a rant about what a terrible president he was. The doctor thought Mom was insightful regarding politics and I was wrong about her condition. And all she said was, "Oh, him!"

One woman in her nineties was sent to a specialist who was a recent immigrant. He was highly regarded in the medical community, but the patient could not understand what he was saying to her. She was perfectly alert; the doctor's accent, however, was too much for her. The patient tried to stay with him because she felt if she didn't she would be discriminating against someone from another country and didn't want to do that. It was clear, however, that she could not grasp his explanations about test results and his instructions to her. The family encouraged her to find another physician whom she could easily understand, and she ultimately did. The patient's needs have to come first.

I read of a spouse who was glad to learn that the trained professionals at elder daycare became as angry at her husband's incessant questions as she did. If you find a facility like this, please grab your loved one and run away as fast as you can. Yes, the constant questions annoy you because you deal with it 24 hours a day. However, trained professionals should NEVER be angry with a dementia patient.

CHAPTER TEN

COPING

Fatigue makes cowards of us all.

-Gen. George S. Patton

OCCASIONALLY MOM would wake up in the middle of the night and think it was daytime. She couldn't tell that it was dark out and she wandered around the house. That usually woke me. When she didn't find anyone to talk to she usually went back to bed. If not, I would get up and guide her back to her bedroom.

One morning she walked into my bedroom at about 2 AM. I was asleep, but she flipped on the light switch, which immediately woke me. She casually asked me what I was doing. I explained it was nighttime and that I had been sleeping; then I put her back to bed. Incidents such as these made it harder and harder to get a full night's sleep.

Lack of sleep makes it much harder to deal with even the littlest problems. The fatigue from being a caregiver 24/7 adds to the problem

Mom and Dad both visited the bathroom at night, as you might expect. One night, however, Mom became disoriented. Again, because of her poor vision, she couldn't figure out where she was. I found her in the kitchen, sitting on a wooden chair, half asleep, and peeing. She had been looking for the bathroom and she thought she was on the toilet. She was never incontinent and that was the only accident she ever had. Fortunately, a wooden chair and tile floor is very easy to clean up. She was upset, though, because she could not reorient herself to figure out where she was.

* * *

Dad had at least one doctor's appointment each month. Eventually, I felt that I could not face another doctor's visit. I asked my sister to take Dad to his appointment. To my relief, she agreed. As the time for the appointment drew closer, she mentioned that I had to go with because she didn't know enough about Dad's condition. I never did get a rest from going to see doctors and getting bad news. Even when the news was good—that he was no worse or a little better—the doctors always made a point of saying everyone dies sometime and it can happen at any moment. I couldn't get that thought out of my mind: that this might be the moment he dies, or this moment, or this moment.

I felt that I could not face another doctor's visit.

Family members accused me of a being a 'control freak.' They were right; I did control everything in my parents' lives. I didn't have a choice. But being called a control freak hurt.

Mom kept losing the sash to her bathrobe. She had several robes, so when she lost the belt to the first one, I took one from another robe. That one disappeared, too, so I gave her the belt from another bathrobe. That also disappeared. I checked the robe pockets, the closet, the floor of the closet. I gave her the belt from my robe and finally stumbled upon the answer. I watched as Mom took off her robe prior to going to bed. She casually took the makeshift belt out of the belt loops and then carefully rolled it into a ball. Then she carefully put the belt in the back of a dresser drawer underneath her scarves. I found all the missing belts there in pile. Apparently, Mom was just being neat!

I would encourage you to find the humor in situations like this and enjoy it to make it easier to cope.

Then, Mother lost the toilet paper holder. Just the rod that goes through the roll. She came out of the bathroom holding the roll of TP. She could not figure out what happened. She had not flushed the toilet and it wasn't in there. And she swore it happened while she was sitting on the potty. That happened many years ago and we never did find the darn thing—not even in the catch basin. Fortunately, we could easily buy a replacement.

Mother lost the toilet paper holder.

Mom also lost her false teeth. She always had them in her mouth—she only had an upper plate. When she went to bed, she put them in a special little bowl on her dresser; the same bowl for decades. Then one day I looked at her and she didn't have her teeth. She had no idea how she could have lost them. We couldn't find them anywhere—not even in the catch basin (are you detecting a trend here?) A few days later, my sister stopped over. She pulled over a chair in the kitchen and sat down. She suddenly said she found the teeth. I thought she was kidding because she hadn't moved, she just sat there saying, "I found them, I found them."

She HAD found them. The kitchen table was a pedestal style and had four "feet" radiating out from the center post. The teeth were under one of the "feet." I had been on my hands and knees looking for them, but never found them. My sister, though, was on an angle where she could see the teeth. Apparently, Mom had taken the teeth out of her mouth, wrapped them in a handkerchief, and put them in her robe pocket. They slid out when she was seated at the table. She NEVER took her teeth out except to put them in the bowl at night or to clean them in the bathroom. I could not have anticipated this one! You HAVE to laugh.

* * *

Sometimes caregivers have to manage by crisis. One time, my father was released from the hospital and I was prepared to take him home. I learned at the time of his discharge that he was going to be on a very strict diet. I brought him home, and he was hungry and needed lunch immediately. I had nothing in the house that fitted his new, very restricted diet. Compare this with bringing home a new baby. One has had time—months—to prepare for the arrival. I'm mentioning this because some of the literature about aging is written as if one has a great deal of time to prepare for every contingency. In real life, many things have to be handled on an emergency basis.

These little things become problems to cope with. We had a block party where we were supposed to eat at noon, but by 1 p.m., the food was nowhere near being ready. Dad was looking forward, to it but he had to eat very regularly. I had to scramble to find lunch for Dad. They finally served about 2 p.m., too late for us to participate. A block party is an all-volunteer event, so it was very hard for them to serve on time. I should have realized that and not counted on them for Dad's lunch.

The doctor decided to remove a small growth from my father's face. I had been squeamish in the past, but my new role of caregiver was getting me past that. The nurse told me I had to leave the room. The doctor said, no I should watch. And I did watch him use the scalpel and gently cut away the growth and then stitch up the cut. Instead of becoming squeamish, I found it rather interesting.

* * *

Dad thought Mom could "do better" if she just tried. He believed she was in a fog because she wasn't trying hard enough to stay sharp. As a result, he yelled at her in an effort to get her back to the way she was. Dad didn't do it often, but, occasionally, when a task was beyond her ability, he would shout to "encourage" her. Some who witnessed Dad's outbursts felt he was being abusive, but he was frustrated and saddened that he was "losing" his wife.

Dad thought Mom could "do better" if she just tried.

At that point, I had to deal with Dad's upset as well as with Mom's issues. It was a lot to cope with and because of family dynamics, I couldn't be an impartial observer to all this.

I tried to develop a predictable rhythm to our life together. I mentally prepared myself that one day a week would be a total loss as far as accomplishing anything, because of emergencies. During one bad period, I spent the better part of one day per week in the emergency room with either Dad or Mom or some other family member. Other less life threatening emergencies occurred quite often, so I just had to schedule in one floating day per week where I didn't expect to accomplish any chores.

Because Mom and Dad were on low-salt diets, I "diluted" the store-bought spaghetti sauce with salt-free tomato sauce. I divided the jar of sauce into four containers, using one and freezing the other three. However, Mom suddenly believed she had to make dinner even though she hadn't cooked for several years. She went into the freezer and found the three containers of spaghetti sauce.

> ## Clearly, this wasn't it a big deal, but I found it hard to cope when little things like this kept happening.

When I came into the kitchen, she was defrosting all three to use because one container wasn't enough for the pasta she planned to make. Clearly, this wasn't a big deal, but I found it hard to cope when little things like this kept happening.

* * *

We always made orange juice from a can of frozen concentrate. I bought two cans when they were on sale and put them in the freezer compartment of the kitchen refrigerator. When I went to use them, they weren't there. I assumed we had used them and I simply forgot. I bought another can and put that in the freezer compartment until I had time to make it. When I went to get that, it was gone. I thought I was getting awfully forgetful. Sometime later, I was in the basement and looked into our old refrigerator, which was left over from the time our basement had been used as an apartment. We kept miscellaneous items in it, including soft drinks, and things that were too big to fit in our upstairs refrigerator such as the turkey defrosting for Thanksgiving, or a whole watermelon.

I found the missing orange juice concentrate. Mom had been taking it out of the kitchen freezer and putting it in the basement refrigerator. Unfortunately, she put it in the refrigerator and not the freezer compartment so it had melted and dripped out of the cans. I was not as forgetful as I feared, but I had no idea that Mom was going into the freezer so often, or that she was going downstairs.

Another situation that was potentially much more dangerous also involved the freezer. From time to time, we would have leftovers that had gone bad, often becoming moldy. I would throw the entire container into the garbage can. When I went to take the garbage out to the alley one day, I found Mom going through it. I had never known her to do that before. As I watched, she picked two containers out of the garbage and started to put them into the freezer. I stopped her, but it's possible that if I hadn't caught her I could have taken the container with the spoiled food from the freezer and used it unwittingly.

Fortunately, that never happened; or I like to think that never happened!

As I watched, she picked two containers out of the garbage and started to put them into the freezer.

Mother often went around the house, before and after she had dementia, singing and reciting poetry. Toward the end of her life, she often recited Henry Wadsworth Longfellow's Revolutionary War poem, "The Midnight Ride of Paul Revere," or at least the beginning part:

> *Listen my children and you shall hear*
> *Of the midnight ride of Paul Revere,*
> *On the eighteenth of April, in Seventy-five;*
> *Hardly a man is now alive*
> *Who remembers that famous day and year.*

Mom died on the eighteenth of April, a fact that I find amazing—and a little unsettling.

CHAPTER ELEVEN

THINGS TO TRY

Most of the important things in the world have been accomplished by people who have kept on trying when there seemed to be no hope at all.

-Dale Carnegie

CREATIVE AND FLEXIBLE! That's been my theme throughout the book. Here are some things I tried.

I bought a lightweight folding wheelchair that I could get in and out of the car, if necessary. Neither parent NEEDED a wheelchair, but Dad had severe arthritis in his knees. Toward the end of his life, he walked with a cane, but he couldn't go more than about 100 feet without becoming tired and achy. With the chair, I could take him for walks. He especially loved it when his two-year-old great grandson rode on his lap. Dad pointed out birds and flowers, colorful leaves and Halloween decorations. One day, at the end of his life, he suddenly became very weak. I took him to the doctor using the wheelchair. He had to go to the hospital and I used the chair for that, too. I was so glad we had it available. Since then, I have loaned it to various people who suddenly needed a wheelchair.

* * *

I'm sorry not to be politically correct, but I feel we need "TV programs for dummies." We have children's programming but people with dementia could benefit from some programs tailored to them that are not overwhelming. Mom watched the news at 10 p.m. every night. She was especially interested in what the weather would be the next day. A typical weather forecast would include information about the entire United States before a discussion of local weather. A typical report might include the information that the Rockies are having a snowstorm, but locally we're having a sunny day with high temperatures nearing 70 degrees. I asked Mom what the weather was going to be after she heard one of these programs.

"Sunny," she would say.

Then she quickly added, "No, there's a snowstorm; no it will be in the seventies—oh, I don't know!"

She was agitated after every broadcast remembering bits but realizing they didn't make sense when she tried to put them together. She could have understood if someone had simply stated it would be sunny and 70.

> Then she quickly added, "No, there's a snowstorm; no it will be in the seventies—oh, I don't know!"

I tried using children's programming—after all, it couldn't hurt for Mom to review her numbers and letters on Sesame Street—but even though her mind was failing making her SEEM childlike, she had no interest in childish things.

* * *

Many programs were recommended to us by Mom's visiting geriatric nurse. For example, legally blind individuals can receive books on tape for free from the Library of Congress.

The most rewarding part of most tasks is finishing it. When teaching a child to put on socks and shoes and then tying the shoes, therefore, the child feels more successful if all he does is finish the bow rather than if all he does is put on the sock. Teaching a task backwards; that is, how to finish the bow first, then all the steps to making a bow, then how to get the shoe on the foot, and finally putting on the sock, is the most satisfying to the child. This holds true for people with dementia as well. If the person can do only one thing, try to make sure it is the last step of the task for a greater sense of accomplishment.

* * *

> # I bought a box of animal crackers and intentionally put it away in the cabinet expecting Mom to find it.

My mother was always looking around the kitchen for a snack. I bought a box of animal crackers and intentionally put it away in the cabinet expecting Mom to find it. She did find it herself and enjoyed eating the cookies. I could have simply given her something to eat, but she seemed to enjoy looking for a snack and finding something appropriate. I suspect she thought she was "putting one over" on me. Perhaps she felt she was caring for herself without asking for help. I don't know what drove that behavior, but this worked well with her.

* * *

Mom and Dad didn't have any serious incontinence issues. After having given birth, my mother would drip one drop if she sneezed or laughed. When she was much older, there would be one drop during the night, which would wake her up, and she would go to the bathroom. She was very "old school," so she used a piece of white cotton from a bed sheet as a pad in her underwear.

This cloth worked well, but when she ran out of old bed sheets, I gave her menstrual pads or liners instead. They were the best. Then I tried the absorbent pads designed for those who are incontinent. The pads wick away the moisture and let the wearer feel dry all the time. These pads were absolutely NO help for my mother—they were worse than nothing. That little drop of moisture she used to feel which woke her and sent her to the bathroom was gone. So, not feeling wet, she kept sleeping until she did have a major accident with bed-wetting. I am sure the pads are great for some, but for anyone with diminished capacity who needs a "little message" in the form of a drop of moisture, they are counterproductive.

* * *

One elderly lady was supposed to eat a banana every day. Unfortunately, near the end of her life, she couldn't bear the smell of bananas. Previously she had gotten her daily banana by having it cut up on top of her morning cereal. The problem was solved by cutting up the banana and putting it in the bottom of the bowl with the cereal and milk poured on top. This was an easy fix for an annoying problem, but one that took a certain amount of creativity and flexibility.

> ## When Dad got a hearing aid, he said he hated how things sounded. I tried it. Everything did sound tinny.

I would encourage you to try to understand what someone is going through as much as much as possible. When Dad got a hearing aid, he said he hated how things sounded. I tried it. Everything did sound tinny. Even worse, I could hear vibrations that I never heard before. Every clank of a pot or utensil was followed by very annoying vibrating sounds. I felt the more I understood what my parents were experiencing, the better I was as a caregiver.

* * *

Childcare experts tell parents to have toys available to young children that are too advanced for them because you never know what day the child will be ready for something more challenging. If they're available, they will play with them when they're ready. Similarly, with elderly people, try to have a variety of activities available.

I've said this before but I'll repeat: You must come to all these projects sideways—just have them around. It's much too stressful for the patient to be handed a game. It seems like you're challenging them to prove they're okay.

* * *

> ## Dad was not home, Mom was oblivious, and the family car was missing.

I never had a problem with either parent wandering off. However, one day I went shopping with my sister in her car. When she brought me home, Dad was not home, Mom was oblivious, and the family car was missing. I was frantic because Dad didn't just take off at that point in his life, although he did still have a driver's license. As it turned out, he left just a moment before we came home. After dropping me off, my sister spotted his car going down the street and followed him. Dad went to his barber. He got there and came home with no problem and my sister was able to phone me and tell me where he was.

* * *

Mom's blindness caused all sorts of problems—for example, we had to keep keeping the floors clear of everything so it was safe for her to walk anywhere. She could walk into an open door that was usually closed or into a closed door that was usually open. I bought bright yellow and neon orange tape to put on edge of doors, at eye level. These were the doors that had to be opened occasionally. Mom wouldn't expect them to be open and could easily bump into them. She probably would be able to see the tape even though she couldn't see the dark brown wood of the doors. We kept doors that should be closed, closed (bedroom and attic doors) as much as possible and the open doors open, too (we kept the bathroom door open unless it was occupied), but sometimes they had to be used and it might be just as Mom was walking by.

CHAPTER TWELVE

DAD

Every day, in every way, I'm getting better and better.

-Émile Coué

THIS WAS DAD'S favorite saying, and he often told me I should repeat it to myself and believe it, and I think he believed it as well.

Snow Shoveling Fear

Because of his heart condition, my father was strictly forbidden to shovel snow. However, he still wanted to shovel because he felt it was his responsibility and too much work for me. As a result, I had to be certain to be awake at daybreak when it was snowing because my father might get up early and shovel the first thing in the morning. At one point, I was able to work part time. I lived with the fear that it might snow while I was away, and he might start shoveling before I could get home to do it. He thought he was doing a good thing, but it actually caused me more worry. I never came up with a good way to handle this.

The Thunderstorm

I awoke one morning to a violent thunderstorm. Mom was in bed asleep but I could not find Dad. I went through the house, attic to basement, with no luck. Then I remembered that Dad had mentioned the day before that the gutters really needed cleaning. I went outside and, sure enough, Dad was on the aluminum ladder cleaning the gutters in the terrible downpour with thunder roaring and lightning flashing. It was the first time I ever spoke to him this way, but I said something along the lines of, "You're an idiot, get inside, now!"

83

To my amazement (and gratification), he did get inside immediately. I think he was torn between wanting to stop and his work ethic that mandated that any time you decide to do a chore, you do it no matter what. This was a clear role reversal moment when I had to be the parent because Dad was acting like a child by not acting safely.

"You're not my mother."

"No, I'm the person who has to take care of you when you're sick."

After that, I occasionally gave specific orders to my father. He was about to go outdoors one cold, rainy day without a warm coat or anything to keep dry. He never did that before—he would, if anything, err on the side of caution. I told him he had to dress more appropriately. That's when he said, "You're not my mother."

And I, who had always been a bit intimidated by my father, said, "No, I'm the person who has to take care of you when you're sick."

That sentence just came out. I didn't mean to say it—I didn't realize I ever thought it. But after that, Dad was much more aware about how his actions affected me.

Driving

When Dad was in his late eighties, I thought it was time he gave up driving. He wasn't driving badly, although the heavy Chicago traffic was a challenge. Dad was very hard of hearing, however, and he did have a heart problem that could flare up at any moment. I didn't know how to approach the problem. The next time he needed to be tested for his driver's license, he didn't do too badly, although he began the test trying to start the engine, which was already running. He couldn't hear it. The examiner took me aside and said he didn't know what to do, he's okay, but he didn't even know the motor was running! I asked him to please turn down his application for renewal. I was lucky—Dad took losing his license well. I know many people do not. Dad could go anywhere he wanted at any time because I was there to be the driver 24/7. Dad actually did "drive" two times after losing his license. The first was when we were in a parking lot and someone parked illegally, partially blocking me in. I couldn't maneuver the car to get out of the space.

I was lucky—Dad took losing his license well.

Dad said, "Let me," and proceeded to pull the car out of the parking space without touching the other vehicle.

The other time was when I was trying to parallel park the car. I don't get any practice because we live in an area with plenty of room to park: sometimes our car was the only one parked on our side of the street.

This time Dad just said, "Move over," and I got out and let him maneuver the car again into position, so easily. I began to wonder if the wrong person had given up driving.

In the Kitchen

At one point while caring for my parents, I came down with the stomach flu. I made myself the only thing in the house I could eat—gelatin.

Dad saw it and wanted some. I explained that I made it for myself and it was the only thing I could eat. He got into this really strange mood, and said it was his house, and he guessed he could eat whatever he wanted, so he ate my gelatin. I had to go without eating that day because there was nothing else my stomach could tolerate. That seemed like a sacrifice beyond any call of duty, but I don't know how else I could handle it once Dad got into that peculiar mindset—which, fortunately, was pretty rare.

My own personal definition of heck came later that day. I still had to make dinner, which happened to be fried chicken. The odor of frying chicken was almost intolerable.

Frustration

The three of us, Mom, Dad, and I did get into each other's way a little bit. My favorite bit of frustration was when I dried all the dishes and stacked them on the counter. Then I walked over to the cabinet where they belonged and opened the doors. I picked up the big stack of dishes, went back and turned to put them into the cabinet just in time to see Dad closing the cabinet door. It bothered him to see doors or drawers left open but really, leaving it open for ten seconds while I put the dishes in should not be a problem!

Dad's younger brother died almost a year before Dad died. At the cemetery, Dad asked me if that was the actual casket with Uncle Robert really in it. He had a hard time wrapping his head around the concept of losing his baby brother, even though mentally he was otherwise pretty sharp.

Pain

At one point after Mom had died, Dad was being crabby to the point of being mean to me. I asked him about it and didn't get an answer. I persisted, and he finally blurted out that there was blood when he "went to the bathroom." He was very shaken up and thought he was dying, but after a little more discussion, I realized that his hemorrhoid problem had returned. A visit to the doctor proved I was right. I wish he would have confided in my sooner rather than being so nasty, and worried, for those few days.

Sleeplessness

> "You were in bed for six minutes, don't you think you should give it a little more time before roaming around?" I asked, trying not to sound aggravated.

Dad suffered from insomnia and often left his bed to sleep on the living room couch for a while. One night I heard him going from one room to another, but thought nothing of it. He returned to his bedroom. Six minutes later, he was back on the couch. Yes, I timed him. I went out to the living room.

"What's wrong?" I asked.

"I was in bed, but I couldn't sleep," Dad replied

"You were in bed for six minutes, don't you think you should give it a little more time before roaming around?" I asked, trying not to sound aggravated.

Dad was stunned, "Six minutes! I thought I was in bed an hour and couldn't sleep!"

I rubbed his back while he was on the couch and he quickly fell asleep—and stayed asleep. Sometimes his insomnia and grumpiness were the result of mild aches and pains.

The Fall

Unknown to me, Dad was outside after a heavy snowfall. He had a ladder against the house and was trying to brush the snow off the roof before the roof was damaged. I was indoors and thought I heard my name off in the distance. For a moment it seemed almost like someone was nearby and whispering my name. I quickly realized it had to be Dad calling me from outside. I ran out, fully dressed but without a coat—and only bedroom slippers on my feet. I found Dad lying in the snow where he had fallen from the ladder. He hit an evergreen first and the branches cushioned his fall. Still, he couldn't get up because he was tangled in the shrubbery.

The first thing he said to me was, "Go back inside and put on boots and then come back."

> # And he specifically told me to ignore his screams of pain.

I complied. I was able to get him up, but he had hurt his back and he had spasms. He tried living with the pain for a day. However, he woke up stiff and unable to move out of bed the next morning. Dad called to me and asked me to grab his hand and pull him up—and he specifically told me to ignore his screams of pain. Clearly, his back was not getting better so I had to call an ambulance. The EMTs got Dad into the ambulance without him screaming.

Neatness

All my life Dad insisted on neatness. We were not allowed to gouge out a knife full of peanut butter; we had to scrape off layers so that the surface was always level and neat. And if you made a mistake writing, and you were angry with yourself, and wanted to crumple up that piece of paper—forget it. Paper was to be folded neatly before being discarded in the wastebasket. Carpeting was to be vacuumed daily and each section had to be gone over five times. As he got older, he mellowed and didn't care about such things. He even suggested I worked too hard with housework, and should occasionally skip vacuuming or whatever chore I might be working on at that moment.

A Great-Grandson

As I've explained, our family consisted of Mom and Dad, my sister, and me. Dad expected to have a son but never did. He made a point of teaching his daughters how to make minor repairs around the house. As he worked, one of us assisted him. We learned the basics of landscaping, carpentry, plumbing, electrical work, and the repair of appliances. He took us fishing, too. Eventually he had one grandchild, also a girl. Then, when he was 91, Dad became a great-grandfather—to a boy. The boy, Ethan, was born after we lost Mother. I believe, without Ethan, Dad would have died much sooner. His new great-grandson lived across the street and Dad saw him almost every day. He was crazy about the baby—partly, I think, because he finally had a boy in the family, partly because he always loved kids, but mostly because of his grief at losing Mom.

> The cardiologist's reply surprised me. He said, "It's okay if he lifts Ethan, because that's love."

Because of my Dad's bad heart, he wasn't allowed to lift anything heavy. At Dad's cardiologist appointment, I explained that Dad was breaking that rule; I couldn't stop him from picking up the baby. And the baby was getting bigger every day. The cardiologist's reply surprised me. He said, "It's okay if he lifts Ethan, because that's love."

I'm glad he felt that way, but it wouldn't have mattered if he didn't. Dad couldn't have NOT carried Ethan if his life depended on it—and I was afraid it did.

By the time Ethan was a year and a half, he would ask for his "Grampa" whenever he was in our house. One day, I had to disappointment Ethan; "I'm sorry, honey, Grampa's sleeping."

Ethan stood there as I talked with his Mom, then he suddenly ran as fast as he could into Dad's bedroom. We ran after him trying to catch him before he woke my Dad. I was afraid if Dad was startled awake, it could induce another heart attack. Ethan made it to Dad's bedside before we could catch him, and he slapped his Grampa on the chest to wake him. Dad's eyes flew open and immediately focused on Ethan. They both had big grins on their faces.

This scenario played out many times—I often had to tell Ethan that Grampa was sleeping and he shouldn't wake him. He always said okay—then ran into the bedroom anyway. I fell for it every time. But no harm was done, "because that's love."

CHAPTER THIRTEEN

END OF LIFE ISSUES

When you were born, you cried and the world rejoiced. Live your life so that when you die, the world cries and you rejoice.

- White Elk

AS I'VE MENTIONED, we decided never to send Mom to a nursing home, no matter what. I'm not sure that it is always possible to keep a person at home, even with extra help. We were fortunate, and Mom stayed at home until one day when she didn't feel very well. As we walked with her through the house to go out to the car, she said her legs felt weak. We had to let her down gently on the floor and called 911. She spoke to us a little but by the time the ambulance came, she was unconscious. She died a few hours later in the hospital without regaining consciousness. It was very sudden, which was good for her but shocking for us.

I had talked with Mom about the end of life when she was about 80. She was perfectly lucid at the time, and she said that she felt her life was over but that was okay, she was ready to go, it was enough. That brief conversation was a comfort to me after she was gone.

Contrast that with my father's situation. Dad was having heart problems and was in the hospital. A health care worker came in his room to talk about end of life issues and insisted, despite my vigorous protests, that I leave the room so she could discuss them with my mother. Dad was temporarily "out of it," and these hospital employees only spoke with spouses. Although I was his daughter, and his lawyer, I was not allowed to participate in any discussion. Mom was in advanced stages of dementia at that time, though it wasn't obvious to people who met her casually. I went into the hall and the hospital employee came running out to talk with me having realized my mother wasn't lucid. I did try to explain that Mom was senile, but many people, I found, had to learn that for themselves.

The hospital worker asked me to sign a Do-Not-Resuscitate (DNR) order for my Dad, which would mean they would not use CPR on him if his heart failed. I refused. Dad recovered quite nicely and lived for five or six years after that. As soon as he was well, I told him they wanted me to sign a DNR form indicating that the hospital was not to resuscitate him. I told him I refused.

His reply? "Thank you!"

Unlike my Mom, he was not ready to give up without a fight. I believe there may be a right time for that, but you don't have to be rushed by "bureaucrats" who don't know you and your loved one's situation.

Documents

> # Federal law requires that anyone being admitted to a health care facility be told of the right to make an advance directive.

Various health care decisions should be made in anticipation of the end of life. Some elderly people choose to have a DNR order in place. I would recommend that you contact a lawyer about documents you or another family member might need, such as a power of attorney. The person who has diminished capacity may need a caregiver for his or her property—bank accounts, house, auto, and other assets. Tax returns have to be filed, as well. Only a legally authorized person can make all the necessary decisions. I also recommend creating an inventory list of what the person owns.

Federal law requires that anyone being admitted to a health care facility be told of the right to make an advance directive. (According to Merriam-Webster's online dictionary, an advance directive is a "legal document (as a living will) signed by a competent person to provide guidance for medical and health care decisions (as the termination of life support or organ donation) in the event the person becomes incompetent to make such decisions.")

Illinois[3] law, for example, allows for three types of advance directives: a health care power of attorney; a living will; and a mental health treatment preference declaration. In addition, you can ask your physician to work with you to prepare a DNR order. Other documents may be advisable, too.

As a practical matter, someone should know details of the individual's personal affairs. My father had numerous bank accounts in various banks. He also had several life insurance policies. And even though I helped him with his finances, and Dad was quite organized, I had a hard time tracking down all his assets. Some bank accounts had been closed and insurance policies cashed in. To my surprise, an old certificate of deposit at one bank was still in force. One ancient insurance policy, which my grandmother obtained when Dad was a little boy, was still in effect.

Further, the caregiver may not know all of the person's acquaintances, and a list of those people, perhaps from address books, is good to have, as well. Also, does the individual belong to any organizations, even if he or she is not active?

Medical Decisions

Dad had an enlarged prostate that was beginning to affect his urine flow. He had surgery and the problem was solved.

> The day or two before the surgery, however, I was talking with Dad and he casually said he was not going to have it done.

A few years later, however, he was diagnosed with prostate cancer. The doctor scheduled the surgery and Dad seemed fine with it. The day or two before the surgery, however, I was talking with Dad and he casually said he was not going to have it done. This was a complete 180 for Dad. He always followed the doctors' suggestions. I called our family practitioner and explained.

"Of course, he intends to have the surgery," the physician replied. "Put him on the phone."

Dad spoke to him for a few minutes and then handled the phone back to me. The doctor had to admit that Dad was too upset to have the surgery. Fortunately, within a week or two, Dad said he was willing to go through with it.

The plan, since Dad was well into his eighties, was to remove his testes. The surgery went well, and he was only in the hospital one day, then sent home. The doctor planned to have a nurse come to our house every day to clean the incision. Then he decided that Dad would be too embarrassed to have a nurse do it. My mother was at home but no longer competent.

"I'll teach you what to do," the doctor said to me, refusing to accept my argument that I really couldn't. Really.

So, there was Dad, lying on his back in his bed, naked. Not a sight I had ever seen before. In order to clean the incision, his penis had to be out of the way. If you think I could touch my dad's penis, think again. If you think I could say the word penis to my father, think again.

"Lift yourself up," I commanded Dad.

He dutifully raised himself up onto his elbows.

"No," I said, pointing to his nether region, "lift your SELF up."

Dad got the message.

> "I'll teach you what to do," the doctor said to me, refusing to accept my argument that I really couldn't. Really.

I removed the gauze and braced myself to clean the wound as I had been taught. But the strangest thing happened. Suddenly, it wasn't my father; it was an interesting challenge. If I did it correctly, I would be helping to restore Dad to health. I did as I had been told, then applied the gauze. From that point on, as I cleaned the incision and monitored the remarkable healing each day, I was unable to think that this was Dad, and only saw the amazing ability of the human body to repair itself.

> "Let God make the decision."

Dad told me that when faced with extreme medical issues, get the best medical advice you can, do what the doctors recommend, and "let God make the decision." He wasn't concerned that he might die; he believed it was God's choice. However, he wasn't about to hasten his own death by making unwise choices. In fact, one procedure that was recommended for his heart had about an 80% chance of success but a 20% chance that he would die during the operation. The doctor was not certain if he should take that risk or not, but if he didn't, Dad's health would definitely decline. I explained this to my father. He wanted to do it—there wasn't a doubt in his mind—and the surgery was scheduled. Then I realized that Dad, being deaf, had misunderstood me. He believed the chance of success was 20%, with an 80% chance of dying. His belief in God making the decision was so strong that the doctor's prediction of a 20% chance of success was good enough for him.

Dad was admitted to the hospital in January 2001. We had gone to the family doctor because he felt very weak. In fact, Dad couldn't walk and I had to use the wheelchair. The night before we went to the doctor was very bad. Dad had been able to walk to the bedroom and sat, really collapsed, on the foot of the bed. When it was clear that he wasn't going to get enough strength to move, he decided to go to bed for the night. He could lie down, but his legs dangled over the foot of the bed. Dad didn't have the strength to drag himself up toward the head of the bed. I tried dragging him up as best I could, but it's a very awkward position to maneuver in. Dad was comfortable enough and went to sleep.

The next morning I was able to get him into the wheelchair and I had relatives help get him down the stairs and into the car. The appointment went okay and we came home. (Fortunately, these same relatives that helped were able to have lunch with us, one of Dad's favorite meals—from McDonald's. We couldn't have known it but it was our last meal together.) He was strong enough to sit at the table for a little while and then went to bed.

> # I asked if this was his final illness and was reassured that it was not.

Although it was a Saturday, I got a call late that afternoon from the doctor: get Dad to the hospital immediately. I told Dad; he didn't want to go, but I took him anyway. Was it the right choice? He never came home again. Would it have been better to follow his wishes and let him stay home?

I asked if this was his final illness and was reassured that it was not.

I learned that his problem was a low platelet count. Platelets are in the blood and they help it to clot. Dad was beginning to have bruises on his body. It was about to be a long few weeks in the hospital.

Dad received transfusions of platelets, but his count remained much, much too low. Blood test after blood test failed to help with a diagnosis. He got stronger; he got weaker. Then the doctors decided he was terminal. We stopped his heart medication because there was no point in taking it. Then they thought he was not terminal and they reinstated his heart medicine. He had some kind of kidney failure and he was terminal. The kidney specialist said it could be easily treated and he did treat Dad. Double amounts of blood were drawn so it could be sent to two labs. Dad endured full body X-rays that pained him greatly. The decision was made to take a bone marrow sample. I was told it was painless; I was told it was quite painful.

Then the diagnosis based on the bone marrow sent to the Mayo Clinic came: leukemia.

This was a time of frustration and guilt for me. Dad didn't have an appetite, so I brought him a chocolate milkshake. He didn't have the strength to suck on the straw and spooning it into his mouth wasn't working either. I was told about a special spoon that has a hypodermic type plunger that almost injects the food well into the mouth. I brought that the next day, but too late. Dad was past being able to swallow.

> "That isn't possible," the resident told me, "we don't want to give painkillers because they mask the symptoms."

Dad was in some pain; he had the type of leukemia, AML, which can be horribly painful, and he was given a couple of days to live, maximum. When the resident came in to check on Dad, I asked for something for his pain. He couldn't take anything orally, but it could be given intravenously.

"That isn't possible," the resident told me, "we don't want to give painkillers because they mask the symptoms."

I looked at him and the wild thought went through my mind that he specifically intended to torture my father. I know how irrational that sounds, but I couldn't understand his thinking. I asked him to step outside.

"Do you know his diagnosis?" I asked.

"Yes, it's very sad that he only has a few days to live," came the reply.

Then why would it be important that his symptoms not be masked?

I spoke with our family practitioner and he ordered a morphine drip. Several hours passed before it was brought into the room. Soon after it was begun, Dad, who had been restless, fell asleep. They sent me home and I went because I knew the next night I would be staying around the clock to be with him; I didn't want him to die alone. But sometime around 5 a.m., he slipped away and I got THE phone call. Dad had died alone. I don't think he ever woke up from when he fell asleep from the morphine. I didn't ask.

Dad had died alone.

---

* * *

Dr. Barry Reisberg[4] suggested, in 1982, a scale of seven stages into dementia, particularly Alzheimer's. The first is normalcy, next is forgetfulness, the third definite problems with memory. In the fourth, the memory loss increases. At level five, patients need some assistance. In six, a patient can forget the name of his or her spouse and needs help dressing. Delusional, obsessive and anxiety symptoms appear. At the seventh level, the patient often cannot speak and has no control over his or her body.

I would categorize my mother as being in the equivalent of the sixth stage for a long time. Often this stage includes incontinence, but Mother didn't have this issue. She couldn't remember family members, recent events, or very much of her life.

After the Passing

As you prepare for the loss of your loved one, you have to be ready to let people know about the passing. Are you putting a death notice in the newspaper? Which newspaper? Are there organizations to notify? Out of town friends?

I called my godmother, Harriett, to let her know of Mom's passing. She greeted me by saying she was not doing too well.

"I only had two close friends," Harriett said, "your mother and one other lady. The other lady died two days ago."

Well, what was I to say? "What a coincidence! My mother died within 24 hours of your other best friend."

Of course not. When she asked to speak with Mom, I told her she was weak and she was asleep. My plan was to tell her Mother was getting weaker and weaker, and eventually tell her that Mother died. I was trying to gauge when Harriett was strong enough to hear the news. It turned out that Harriett died before I had a chance to tell her of Mom's passing.

I like to think that even though I lied, I did the right thing. This further illustrates how a caregiver has to be creative and flexible. And that no book can prepare you for your unique challenges.

> # I like to think that even though I lied, I did the right thing.

* * *

My mother and father had wills, but their overall attitude about dying was that it was something that did not bear thinking about. It was inevitable, yes, but better to ignore it until forced to deal with it. So when my mother passed away in the hospital, Dad and I had to find a place to bury her. Our first thought was the cemetery where her mother and siblings were. (I'd like to mention here that my grandmother purchased her own grave well in advance of her old age. In fact, she bought, I think, six, which is why some of her children are around her.) We quickly found lots quite close to my grandmother, so it wasn't too difficult a job to find a final resting place for Mom. However, we hadn't been prepared, and it was hard to perform this task while grieving.

When organizing the funeral itself, remember to contact the organizations that were important in the person's life. Dad had served in WWII, so the funeral director contacted the Navy for me. Navy personnel participated in the service and provided a flag for his coffin. It was a very moving service. Representatives from all Dad's groups, his union, lodge, and the American Legion, attended as well as relatives from his and Mother's side of the family. Each provided a pallbearer for Dad. Somehow, that was very comforting to me.

CHAPTER FOURTEEN

SACRIFICES

Honor thy father and thy mother that thy days may be long upon the land which the Lord thy God giveth thee.

-Exodus 20:12 (King James Version)

PERHAPS THE GREATEST SACRIFICE in caring for my parents and living with them was that I had no safe haven. I had no place to go for peace and quiet. No place to go to get away from it all. No place to go to be comfortable. No place to recharge and unwind. And it felt like I had no home.

As I mentioned before, I had tried working. Getting away for a while, even to work, was a much-needed respite. The schedule for my part time position worked like this: five days a week, I woke up at 5:30 a.m. and left for work at 6:30 AM. I arrived between 7:30 and 8:00. I worked until noon and was home about 1:00 p.m. My parents typically woke up around noon or a little later. I would make lunch when I came home. Then there was the endless round of appointments with doctors, specialists, barbers, dentists, and bank officers; and errands such as grocery and other shopping.

Of course, I needed to interact with Mom and Dad to help them stay as sharp as possible as well as to entertain them. I got to bed about 1:30 a.m. The next day I was up again at 5:30 a.m. I had tried working eight hours a day, three days a week, but that didn't work very well. I had to miss work a lot and eventually gave it up—I wouldn't have tried it at all if my financial situation hadn't been so desperate.

Therefore, when a holiday rolled around and we were invited to someone's home for a celebration, it was a big deal for me. Unfortunately, my father felt bad that he couldn't help the hosts in some way. Therefore, he always insisted that I volunteer to help the hostesses in the kitchen. They usually accepted my offer of help, darn them! I vividly remember working alone in the kitchen washing dishes one Christmas, listening to everyone else opening their gifts in the living room.

I didn't go to a restaurant, movie, concert, play, or other entertainment, for 15 years. I did go to doctor's appointments for myself and to counseling to help me cope with my parents. Since this was years before the Internet, I felt isolated. Don't let this happened to you—isolation is very stressful. You're not helping yourself, and you're not helping your loved one. In fact, Leeza Gibbons who founded Leeza's Place for family caregivers lists "Do Not Isolate" as one of her ten commandments for caregivers. (See Leeza's website for all the commandments at http://www.leezasplace.org/ten_comm.html.)

I didn't go to a restaurant, movie, concert, play, or other entertainment, for 15 years.

I missed one call for an interview because I was in an ambulance with my dad on the way to the ER. My sister had stayed behind to lock up the house before meeting us at the hospital and took the phone call. I never did get back to the interviewer because Dad had a prolonged stay in the hospital. Once, when Dad was in the hospital, I was especially glad for my sister's presence, as things were not going well. Unfortunately for me, she had a job interview and had to leave. I so envied her that she could take off like that, and wished I had support as I learned the bad news about Dad's condition. It couldn't be helped, though, because my sister wasn't working at the time and needed a job.

In the following section, I complain about a certain lack of support. At least that's how it felt. Afterwards I realized that all the resistance I experienced from friends and family came from their grief. I recommend that you put yourself first, and do what you need to do for you. It's on me that I didn't go to the spa or have the photographs I wanted as I discuss below.

I recommend that you put yourself first, and do what you need to do for you.

I took Mother's sudden death very hard. She had been examined one week to the day before she died and pronounced physically fit. I wasn't prepared for her death by heart failure.

Shortly after Mom's death, I was with a small group of acquaintances. One turned to me and said, "Sorry about your loss, but what did you expect, she was old." She shrugged and turned away.

I was stunned at the insensitivity of her comment. Did she think that when a parent reaches a certain age, the children do not love that parent anymore? It was complete nonsense. A few years later, this woman lost her own mother, at least as old as Mom had been. She also took her loss very hard and I knew that now she understood.

I wanted to get away, just for a little while, after the funeral. I was able to have someone who could be with Dad. Finally, rather than an overnight trip, I settled on a day at the spa. I had never been to one, but I thought a massage and whatever they do at spas would help. Foolishly, I mentioned it to family members. I was asked where I would go. I told them of a place I had in mind.

"You don't want to go there; my friend went and didn't like it," I was told.

Another place was judged too expensive. Objections were raised at all my ideas.

I didn't go anywhere. I didn't have even an hour respite.

I think I listened to them because I was so worn down with caregiving and grief that I couldn't stand up for myself. And maybe they were right: maybe they were truly concerned that I was too fragile to risk going anywhere that might possibly treat me poorly.

> It seemed to me in some illogical way, that as soon as I finished the last note, Mom would really be gone.

We sent thank you notes to everyone who signed the guest book at the wake and funeral. I did them over several days. I was about to write the last one when I suddenly couldn't. I walked outside. It seemed to me in some illogical way, that as soon as I finished the last note, Mom would really be gone. I knew she was gone, of course, but while I was dealing with the wake and funeral, it wasn't completely over. I can't explain it, but the last note made the loss real on a completely different level.

I went inside and wrote the note.

After Mom's death, I put her picture in a special frame. I chose a photo from when I was young—when she looked as I always pictured her.

Younger family members complained, "That doesn't look like her."

It looked exactly like her. Was her. Mom. I meekly put the photo away.

Mother's death had hit me like a physical blow and I had found myself walking hunched over. As time went on, I thought I was starting to do better. More than a month later, I was in a department store and was surprised to realize that I was feeling almost normal that day. Then I passed a full-length mirror. I didn't realize it was there, and when I turned I found myself gazing at a stranger. No, it was me! I was shocked. I was bent over (I was sure I was ramrod straight) and my face looked pinched with grief. I looked 20 years older than my age. A good reality check for me—I had a long way to go.

> # Mother's death had hit me like a physical blow and I found myself walking hunched over.

I've heard of friends and neighbors showering a grieving family with food—casseroles, baked goods, the cooks' specialties. That would have been wonderful but didn't happen after either of my parent's deaths. Please don't have any expectations. People can only do what they can.

My father's death was very hard because it meant living alone in my parents' house with my parents' things. How the house creaked! I really had a hard time sleeping now. I could still hear the sounds I had previously attributed to Dad's movement. I wanted more interaction with my family, but I guess I was too needy.

"You have to learn to live alone," I was told.

My brother-in-law passed away two years after my mother's death and two years before my father's. My sister put together a board with pictures of him for the wake. I was invited to contribute one. In the last years of his life, he adopted a funky hairstyle that I, well, hated. I chose a photo from a few years earlier where he was looking handsome.

Younger family members complained, "That doesn't look like him."

My photo was not part of the collage.

I will remember Mom and my brother-in-law as I choose.

CHAPTER FIFTEEN

YOU

If you are seated next to someone who might need some assistance, such as…an individual with limited physical or mental capabilities…you should put your own mask on first, then breathe normally as you assist the other person. That way, if the other struggles, you will have a steady flow of oxygen as you fight the person to get their mask on.

-Kevin Coffey

WE HAVE ALL HEARD, or heard about, the above airplane emergency instructions: we must take care of ourselves first before we can help anyone else. This is as true with caregiving as it is with oxygen masks.

This book is written from the point of view of a younger person taking care of a parent or other elder. Of course, often it is a spouse caring for a spouse. Or a sibling for a sibling. These situations create entirely different emotional issues. You "expect" to lose some one a generation older, but not so with someone approximately the same age.

You may feel grief as you watch someone decline or slip away. Emotions may be around the role reversal you're experiencing. Your parent becomes your child. You may have thought of yourself as the weaker person in the relationship and now you have to be the strong one. Maybe you were never comfortable making decisions, but now you have to make them all the time. Throughout this very difficult time, you must care for yourself first. You will be a better caregiver for it.

I wish I could give you ideas for caring for yourself, but I was a complete failure in that area. To some extent, I stopped living my life for 21 years. I still live with the repercussions of my decision as I write this, approximately 10 years after ending my caregiving "career." I started writing the book as a catharsis—when I wondered what kind of life I could have after "losing" ages 30 to 50. I lost the opportunity to marry and have children. And I may never recover financially.

When I did try to care for myself, things often went wrong. One day I felt the need to get out of the house for a little while. My sister and I went for ice cream at a place two blocks from my house. Even though we were gone for less than an hour, I came home to an upset household. Dad had fallen. He never fell before, and I don't know why he did that time. He was in the basement and he just could not get up. Dad had called for my mother to help him, but at first, she didn't hear him. Then she heard him but could not comprehend what he wanted her to do. Finally, she helped him up. Fortunately, he was not hurt at all, but I suffered tremendous guilt for leaving my parents alone for even that short a period, especially for something as frivolous as ice cream.

> # When I did try to care for myself, things often went wrong.

My parents would not consent to having any help in the house other than family members. I might have been able to convince Dad, but Mom would have been too frightened to have strangers in the house. The family doctor and my father's cardiologist agreed that they didn't really need close supervision. Even though I was caring for my parents in the way the doctors recommended, I kept feeling guilty.

I went to counseling to help me cope with my parents. I found it helpful. When Mom died and it was only Dad and me in the house, the dynamics of the situation changed and counseling helped me with that, too. Not all of her advice was useful, though. When Mom died, she recommended I buy a goldfish. A goldfish to replace my mother? Anyway, I had Dad to care for and talk to.

> # I went to counseling to help me cope with my parents.

I hope I have given you enough examples of things that happened to me that you can prepare yourself to expect the unexpected and handle anything that comes your way—without any long-term after effects. Know that the books by medical experts are guides only—your situation could be different. Be creative and flexible in thinking of ways to deal with the issues you face.

I was criticized once by a neighbor I barely knew, at a party at my sister's house. Mom wanted to look at something, and she had to put it right up to her eyes to see it. The neighbor was outraged that we allowed her to live her life with such poor eyesight. Before Mom had dementia, she read the newspaper with it so close to her eyes that newsprint rubbed onto her nose. She said that when she went to bed she could see the threads in the pillowcase clearly enough to count them.

As she aged, Mom went from being extremely nearsighted to becoming legally blind. According to the eye doctor, no glasses could help her. That was not enough for the neighbor who ripped me apart for my "lack of care." I would suggest to every caregiver be prepared for the comments of uninformed strangers, friends, and family. Most of the time the caregiver is complimented on his or her dedication in caring for the loved one, but there are always those who will criticize out of ignorance.

> ## The neighbor was outraged that we allowed her to live her life with such poor eyesight.

Once when Dad was in the hospital but doing well and scheduled to come home, some relatives stopped by. I lit the log in the fireplace and turned around to see them apparently very upset. I asked what was wrong but didn't get a reply.

Finally, the timid response came, "Your dad always did that."

No, he didn't. Sometimes he did, but sometimes I lit it. I didn't know what to do with their distress. Never have a comforting fire in the fireplace unless Dad was there to light it? Was I being callous? After Dad died, would the fireplace never be used again? Was everything he did something sacred that could not be touched by another family member without committing a sacrilege? Their reaction upset me terribly.

> ## The sound triggered a deluge of memories from childhood winters when I would come home to a kitchen warm and fragrant with Mom's cooking.

Sometimes doing something that a loved one "always" did triggers off memories. I was surprised at my emotional response one time while making dinner. We had lost Mom a year or so previously. I was using a certain metal saucepan, and the spoon made a unique clanging noise against that pan. The sound triggered a deluge of memories from childhood winters when I would come home to a kitchen warm and fragrant with Mom's cooking. Bittersweet and totally unexpected.

Planning Your Finances

A new trend is having the non-caregiving family members pay the caregiver for his or her services. A nice idea but not without its pitfalls because of the family dynamics inevitably involved. From what I read, the average pay is for 20 hours per week! What about the caregiver who is there 24/7 and often up during the night? Could any family afford this kind of care?

In my case, I had free room and board while living in my parents' home. They also paid for a portion of some of my expenses—part of my health insurance and auto insurance. However, I put myself in real economic jeopardy. There were two problems for me: I could not work as an attorney. I could work at some temporary part-time jobs, but not at the compensation an attorney is expected to receive. Secondly, I was out of the job market for so long that it was a problem to re-enter the job market. I had expenses that outpaced the small amount I earned. In my situation, I compromised my present and had to live a rather austere life—I remember looking lustfully at a magazine I could not afford—but I also compromised my future ability to provide for myself. It was awful at the time knowing I had spent most of my savings and had lost my peak earning years. At the same time, I knew that if I continued as a caregiver, the end of my financial problems could only end with the death of both my parents.

As I mentioned, my mother died first. During my father's last year of life, I was in a panic most of the time knowing I was almost completely broke. I had to do something, I thought, or I would literally become a bag lady living on the streets. Would it be possible to find a job now and still care for Dad? I began searching for a job again, but Dad's condition worsened. He soon passed away.

> **During my father's last year of life, I was in a panic most of the time knowing I was almost completely broke.**

What a horrible position to be in! After Dad was gone, I shared an inheritance with my sister. This amount was enough to get me through a few years as I tried to become reestablished in the working world. However, it was a tough sell to be hired again. No one should have to be put in that position. It was however, a position I put myself in by choosing to continue to be a caregiver.

My recommendation to any caregiver is do NOT do what I did! Review your personal finances often and make the necessary changes IMMEDIATELY. Do not compromise your entire financial future! Each caregiver has a unique situation so I cannot make any specific suggestions, but do take care of your finances.

I found it very important to allow enough time for activities to reduce my stress. For example, it was physically possible for me to drive to our local grocery store, shop for a few items, and be back within a half hour—if everything went perfectly. Of course, it never did go perfectly, but still I "allowed" myself only thirty minutes for the trip. Finally, I had to make a point of blocking out an hour in my schedule for the errand. Usually I was home in about 45 minutes, which made me feel very good. However, when I expected it to take a half hour and it took 45 minutes, I was stressed. By the simple mental adjustment of expecting the trip to take one hour, I dramatically reduced my stress level.

> **I found it very important to allow enough time for activities to reduce my stress.**

I would recommend having someone stay overnight so you can get some sleep yourself. I had an aunt who stayed over one night, and it was the best sleep I had had in years. Ideally, you want to be away and have someone take over for you, but if you can't do that, this is the next best thing.

If your loved one is in the hospital, be aware that you have the right to hire a private nurse to be with him or her in the hospital. Sometimes a hospital is so understaffed that the patient seems to get adequate care only when family members monitor the situation. In those cases, a night nurse may be helpful.

Many places are available now to provide support to the caregiver. The Internet lists countless resources including Leeza Gibbon's Memory Foundation, <http://www.leezasplace.org>, and the Rosalynn Carter Institute for Caregiving, <http://rci.gsw.edu>.

Help is available through local, state, and federal programs. In May 2010, the Caregiver and Veterans Omnibus Health Services Act of 2010 became law. I had contacted my congressman and senators urging them to vote for this bill. The legislation provides support to family caregivers for certain injured veterans. Eligible caregivers of veterans can receive health care, training, counseling, support and a stipend.

Finally, it doesn't hurt to check in with yourself and decide if your habits are changing in a negative way. For example, are you drinking too much?

CHAPTER SIXTEEN

AFTERWARDS

If they give you lined paper, write the other way.

-William Carlos Williams

I INCLUDED THE ABOVE quotation as a sort of summary of what I've been saying throughout the book. To best care for the elderly, you will have to use your ingenuity—be creative and flexible. Only you know what you're going through and you're in the best position to devise ways to deal with your circumstances. Just don't be so entrenched in your passive role of "child" (or younger generation) that you fail to take charge of your parent's situation (or other elderly person) as soon as it becomes necessary.

After Mom died, Dad lived for three and one half years more. They were married for 66 years and had dated for several years before that—Mom was 20 and Dad 23 when they married—so they really had been together about 70 years.

If it weren't for his great-grandson, Ethan, Dad wouldn't have made it that long. Ethan, born when Dad was 91, was very close to his Grampa. They had an incredible rapport. We had a family photo portrait taken a few months before Dad died. First, we were all photographed together. Then the photographer asked everyone to step into the reception room while he took more photos just of Dad. We were only in the room a moment when Ethan broke away to be with his Grampa. The photographer never got his shots of Dad alone; he had to settle for pictures of Dad holding Ethan. They were inseparable.

* * *

> ## The tests came back after she was gone and the doctor told me that Mom's "brain was calcified."

Mom had tests in the hospital a few days before she passed away. The tests came back after she was gone and the doctor told me that Mom's "brain was calcified." He said that it would not have been surprising if she had been a vegetable. Instead, she was functioning fairly well: her memory was gone but she was able to eat dinner at the table, participate a little bit in the conversation, and then wash the dishes! I would like to take credit for that, but we just don't know why she did as well as she did.

The family doctor wanted to have an autopsy performed on Mom. I did, too, but Dad and other family members were opposed to it so it wasn't done.

* * *

I had become very protective of my mother over the years—so protective that it became a reflex. In fact, right after she died I had this very brief, wild thought: How will she handle Heaven without me to help? I know how crazy it sounds, but it was so hard to stop being the caregiver. For about a year after Mom's death, I found myself putting raisin bread in my shopping cart for her breakfast. Caring for her had become a habit.

> ## Some of these people thought I was lying or exaggerating, and if Mom did any one little thing "normally," they refused to believe she had any issues at all.

Part of my need to protect Mom stemmed from strangers not knowing she had a diminished capacity and expecting too much of her. Most people quickly caught on that she had issues before I had a chance to explain. A few people, though, held her to the highest standards even after being told that Mom had senile dementia and could not function normally. Some of these people thought I was lying or at least exaggerating, and if Mom did any one little thing "normally," they refused to believe she had any issues at all.

I have seen this intolerance, or perhaps more accurately, misunderstanding, with other dementia patients as well. One man with advanced Alzheimer's who needed a full-time paid caregiver spoke harshly to old friends. It wasn't really the patient speaking; of course, it was the dementia. One long-time friend said he couldn't forgive him for his thoughtless comments. I cannot understand how forgiveness can be a problem. The man was long past the time of making any sense when he spoke. I completely understand if old friends find it too painful or upsetting to be around the dementia patient, and, if the friends never want to speak to the patient again, that's fine. However, it is beyond my comprehension how those old friends can refuse to forgive the uncontrollable outbursts of someone in the advanced stage of a terrible disease. Do you have trouble forgiving a stroke victim for not being able to speak clearly? Do you have trouble forgiving an accident victim for not being able to walk quickly with an injured leg? Of course not. However, this is the sort of intolerance the dementia patient and the caregiver have to deal with every day; and that's why I became so protective of my mom. Part of the problem is the person with dementia does have "good days," or "better days." When a friend talks to the person on one of the "good days," he becomes lulled into thinking (or certain in his conviction) that there is no dementia and the harsh comments previously made were intentional insults by a fully functioning adult. This just adds to the problem and the hurt feelings.

Lose Yourself in Your Work

The next unfortunate person who says to me, "Well, when someone you love dies, you should just lose yourself in your work," is going to be punched in the nose.

If your entire day, week, month, year is taken up with caring for someone, that IS your work and you have nothing else in which to "lose yourself." And you probably cannot immediately go out and get a job. Assuming you are emotionally capable, it is still a time consuming process to get a job! I had spent as much time as possible each week doing volunteer administrative work to stay in touch with the real world. Although it was a good outlet for me, it didn't help with finding a job.

…punched in the nose.

As difficult as it may seem, you have to plan for your life after your role of caregiver ends. Just as parents often plan for when they will have an "empty nest" as their youngest child leaves for college, you need to plan, too. What is so difficult is that you probably don't know when the inevitable will happen. It's hard to make specific plans, but anything you can do toward preparing for the future is helpful. I couldn't have guessed how long my parents would live based on their parents' lives. My mother showed signs of senility while still in her sixties. However, HER mother lived to be 87 and was sharp until her last two years, which were after she fell and broke her hip. My father's mother died of cancer in her early 50s and his father died of a heart attack in his early 60s, yet Dad lived to be 93.

Just as parents often plan for when they will have an "empty nest" as their youngest child leaves for college, you need to plan, too.

One day, when my dad was still alive, I was looking at some literature about train trips. Dad asked about it, and I said I would really like to go on a trip like that. He thought that was great...and asked me when I planned to go. I was caught completely off guard. If I were completely honest with him, I would have said that it was something I intended to do after he died. I couldn't say that, of course.

While I was caring for my parents, our local paper reported on a family that lived a few blocks from us. A son was caring for his elderly parents. Apparently, they formed a suicide pact, and all three died together. It's always sad to read about suicide but this hit me particularly hard because they were so physically close as well as in a situation almost identical to mine.

* * *

After you lose someone, you may react in one of many different ways. None of these ways is wrong. My sister was unable to cry for about six months after losing Mother. I was living with Mother, and with her when she died in the hospital. When I came home, I couldn't walk through the door. For some reason it seemed impossible to be in that house knowing she would never be there again. I was okay and able to go in the house after a few minutes of talking with my sister and father. Odd things like this happen. I have had people apologize for being weepy months or years after a loss but I tell them it would be odd NOT to feel anything. By the way, I always wondered: if the loss of someone close to us is a terrible event, why should we EVER feel good about it? We don't. The passage of time makes the hurt much less raw, but loss never becomes a POSITIVE part of our past.

> After you lose someone, you may react in one of many different ways. None of these ways is wrong.

After Dad lost his driver's license, he was dependent on me to take him wherever he wanted to go. He was invited to the occasional brunch or dinner sponsored by organizations he belonged to. The invitations were always "plus one," and since I was driving, I attended these events, too. I became friends with his friends and chatted with the wives. They were older than I was, but considerably younger than Dad. They weren't close relationships, but we exchanged Christmas cards and looked forward to catching up with each other in person.

Then Dad died in January. These friends all attended his funeral and were supportive. The following Christmas, however, I wrote to all of them, as usual, and almost none of them ever wrote back. I had come to think of them as my friends as well as Dad's, and I was surprised and saddened that most of them dropped me like that. It was a time when I needed every friend I could get. Losing contact with so many people all at once was as real a loss as losing Dad. And by losing people who knew him, it was as if I lost another part of him. I could not have anticipated this happening nor how much it hurt. Now I was grieving another loss.

My sister experienced a similar but perhaps greater loss when her husband passed away. The two of them had many friends, couples, which were perhaps more his friends than hers. He was more gregarious than she, and some of the friendships predated her marriage to him. After my brother-in-law passed away, most of the friends "dropped" her. Some of his family members did, too. My sister is a very shy person so it was hard for her to reach out to them, and they didn't reach out to her.

I encourage you to be aware of the people around you to try to be clear about your relationships, and who will be there for you after your loved one is gone. Don't be blindsided by the loss of those you considered to be your friends.

CHAPTER SEVENTEEN

WHAT I THINK IT ALL MEANS

Take no thought for your life, what ye shall eat, or what ye shall drink;
nor yet for your body, what ye shall put on.

-Matthew 6:25 (King James Version)

DO YOU THINK I complained a lot throughout this book? I know I did, so what I say next may surprise you. During the time I was a caregiver, up until today, I have always considered it a privilege to serve. And as much of a sacrifice as it was, I believe that taking care of each other is what families do.

Countless people told me I did I good thing; that my parents were lucky to have me. A surprising number of people confessed to feeling guilty because they went on with their lives not realizing how deteriorated their parents' health had become.

I personally view my journey in caregiving from a spiritual perspective. At first, I was watching Mom with a sense of loss as she declined. She lost her skills one by one. I began to think about the purpose of the life of someone with dementia. What use is this life of a senile patient? In my mother's case, she was enjoying life, loving her family members even though she was uncertain of their names, and she was savoring her meals and coffee. Mom loved music and the sound of birds singing. Yes, the abilities she had as a functioning adult had slowly melted away.

Looking at my mother, near the end of her life:

Could she have held down a job? Of course not.

Could she have gone to a store just a block away? No.

Could she make food for herself? No, in fact, some days she couldn't work the tap to get a drink of water.

Did she know friends and family member? Not usually.

What could Mom do?

She enjoyed her food. A cup of coffee or a cookie would make her smile.

She gave shoulder massages. If she passed Dad or me sitting in a chair she would often, several times a day, rub our backs.

She always remembered my father. She didn't remember who my sister and I were, but she never forgot her husband. She forgot that she married him and thought she was just dating him, but she never forgot the love.

What had she lost?

The mundane. The worldly. She lost interest in clothes and how she looked—and smelled. She lost interest in all possessions. She lost everything that, when you stop to think about it, doesn't really matter in life.

Her life was stripped down to its essence. Here was clarity in her freedom from the mundane.

Love. She could and did love. She was loved.

I don't know if at some level she knew it. But I knew it, and it had a profound effect on me.

Mother was living the purest form of life.

The time when one loses one's faculties is not just a sad end to a life, but an important period of living.

"What is the purpose of this person's life?" I had been asked about other elderly relatives.

"She's not my mom/grandma/aunt anymore; she might as well be dead."

Just because someone cannot see the "use" of an elderly or senile person's life doesn't mean he or she doesn't have a purpose in this world.

Of course, if someone is in extreme pain, cannot speak, and the end is near, it may be time to let go. But still that doesn't mean there isn't a value in that person's life.

This is from one of those emails that are always circulating, author unknown:

An elderly man was in a hurry to have breakfast with his wife, an Alzheimer's patient in a nursing home. He admitted that she had not recognized him for five years. When asked why he visited her every day, he replied,

"She doesn't know me, but I still know who she is."

117

A woman whose mom had Alzheimer's regularly visited her in the nursing home. The mom was not able to communicate; she couldn't do anything more than grunt. But when her daughter visited, the mom's face would light up. The daughter was greeted with the well-remembered smile. She was still Mom.

What is your expectation? If you haven't seen granny in a year and you are remembering what she was like when you were little, are you setting yourself up for a disappointment?

* * *

One night, near the end of Mom's life, Dad and I couldn't make her understand she had to scoot up in bed. She had sat on the side of the bed too close to the foot, so when she lay down, her feet were almost over the end of the mattress. Nothing Dad or I said made sense to her. Slide up, move higher, "scooch" over—she really couldn't understand what we meant. Finally, Dad leaned over her and slid one arm under her thighs and the other under her shoulders. He lifted her just inches off the bed and redeposited her higher in the bed with her head finally on the pillow.

After he slid his arms out, she said in a disappointed voice, "Oh, I thought you were going to kiss me."

I left the room.

* * *

A few days before Dad passed away in the hospital, a nurse had to draw his blood. He ultimately died of leukemia, but at this point, they were still taking a lot of blood samples to determine what was wrong. The nurse could not get the sample and called in another nurse. The second nurse was able to draw the blood but only after several tries.

She sealed the vial, then turned to Dad, saying, "I know I've hurt you. Here's my hand, slap it to get back at me—you'll feel better."

I watched Dad as he took the nurse's hand, brought it up to his face, and kissed it.

ENDNOTES

Never complain. Never explain.

-Katharine Hepburn

KATHARINE HEPBURN may have been correct, but I'm going to explain where I found the information in this book anyway.

[1]*From Chapter Two*

The only book I feel comfortable recommending to you; one whose philosophy I share is, *My Mother, Your Mother: Embracing "Slow Medicine," the Compassionate Approach to Caring for Your Aging Loved Ones,* by Dr. Dennis McCullough. Here's the book's table of contents:

Preface: Slow Medicine
First Things: The Foundation of a New Family Understanding
Overview: Slow Medicine at Eight Stations of Late Life
Chapter 1: Stability "Everything is just fine, dear" -Mom
Chapter 2: Compromise "Mom's having a little problem" -Dad
Chapter 3: Crisis "I can't believe she's in the hospital" -Sister
Chapter 4: Recovery "She'll be with us for a while" -Rehabilitation Nurse
Chapter 5: Decline "We can't expect much more" -Visiting Nurse
Chapter 6: Prelude to Dying "I sense a change in her spirit" -Long Term Care Nurse
Chapter 7: Death "You'd better come now" -Hospice Nurse
Chapter 8: Grieving/Legacy "We did the right things" Brother

Dr. Dennis McCullough
http://www.mymotheryourmother.com/aboutbook.html
Retrieved June 2, 2010

Georgette H. Tarnow

[2]From Chapter Three and Chapter Nine Part One

What Do You See, Nurse? or Crabbit Old Woman

What do you see, nurse...what do you see?
Are you thinking - when you look at me:
"A crabbed old woman, not very wise;
Uncertain of habit with far-away eyes,

Who dribbles her food and makes no reply
When you say in a loud voice 'I do wish you'd try.'"
Who seems not to notice the things that you do
And forever is losing a stocking or shoe;

Who, resisting or not, lets you do as you will
With bathing and feeding, the long day to fill.
Is that what you're thinking, is that what you see?
Then open your eyes, nurse. You're not looking at me!

I'll tell you who I am as I sit here so still.
As I move at your bidding, eat at your will:
I'm a small child of ten with a father and mother,
Brothers and sisters who love one another;

A young girl of sixteen with wings on her feet,
Dreaming that soon a love she'll meet;
A bride at twenty, my heart gives a leap,
Remembering the vows that I promised to keep;

At twenty-five now I have young of my own
Who need me to build a secure, happy home.
A woman of thirty, my young now grow fast.
Bound together with ties that should last.

At forty, my young sons have grown up and gone,
But my man's beside me to see I don't mourn;
At fifty once more babies play 'round my knee
Again we know children, my loved ones and me...

Dark days are upon me, my husband is dead.
I look at the future, I shudder with dread.
For my young are all rearing young of their own,
And I think of the years and the love that I've known.

I'm an old woman now, and nature is cruel.
'Tis her jest to make old age look like a fool.
The body, it crumbles, grace and vigor depart.
There is a stone where I once had a heart.

But inside this old carcass a young girl still dwells,
And now again my bittered heart swells;
I remember the joys, I remember the pain
And I'm loving and living life over again;

I think of the years, all too few, gone too fast
And accept the stark fact that nothing can last;
So open your eyes, nurse, open and see...
not a crabbed old woman. Look closer...see me!

A poem of uncertain provenance, usually attributed to a Phyllis McCormack. The poem is written in the voice of an old woman in a nursing home who is reflecting upon her life. First published in Chris Searle's poetry anthology Elders (Reality Press, 1973).

Wikipedia
http://en.wikipedia.org/wiki/Crabbit_Old_Woman
Retrieved February 7, 2011.

³***From Chapter Thirteen***

STATEMENT OF ILLINOIS LAW ON ADVANCE DIRECTIVES AND DNR ORDERS

You have the right to make decisions about the health care you get now and in the future. An advance directive is a written statement you prepare about how you want your medical decisions to be made in the future, if you are no longer able to make them for yourself. A do not resuscitate order (DNR order) is a medical treatment order that says cardiopulmonary resuscitation (CPR) will not be used if your heart and/or breathing stops.

Federal law requires that you be told of your right to make an advance directive when you are admitted to a health-care facility. Illinois law allows for the following three types of advance directives: (1) health care power of attorney; (2) living will; and (3) mental health treatment preference declaration. In addition, you can ask your physician to work with you to prepare a DNR order. You may choose to discuss with your health-care professional and/or attorney these different types of advance directives as well as a DNR order. After reviewing information regarding advance directives and a DNR order, you may decide to make more than one. For example, you could make a health care power of attorney and a living will.

If you have one or more advance directives and/or a DNR order, tell your health-care professional and provide them with a copy. You may also want to provide a copy to family members, and you should provide a copy to those you appoint to make these decisions for you.

State law provides copies of sample advance directives forms. In addition, this webpage provides a copy of these forms and a copy of the Illinois Department of Public Health (IDPH) Uniform Do Not Resuscitate (DNR) Advance Directive.

Health Care Power of Attorney

The health care power of attorney lets you choose someone to make health-care decisions for you in the future, if you are no longer able to make these decisions for yourself. You are called the "principal" in the power of attorney form and the person you choose to make decisions is called your "agent." Your agent would make health-care decisions for you if you were no longer able to makes these decisions for yourself. So long as you are able to make these decisions, you will have the power to do so. You may use a standard health care power of attorney form or write your own. You may give your agent specific directions about the health care you do or do not want.

The agent you choose cannot be your health-care professional or other health-care provider. You should have someone who is not your agent witness your signing of the power of attorney.

The power of your agent to make health-care decisions on your behalf is broad. Your agent would be required to follow any specific instructions you give regarding care you want provided or withheld. For example, you can say whether you want all life-sustaining treatments provided in all events; whether and when you want life-sustaining treatment ended; instructions regarding refusal of certain types of treatments on religious or other personal grounds; and instructions regarding anatomical gifts and disposal of remains. Unless you include time limits, the health care power of attorney will continue in effect from the time it is signed until your death. You can cancel your power of attorney at any time, either by telling someone or by canceling it in writing. You can name a backup agent to act if the first one cannot or will not take action. If you want to change your power of attorney, you must do so in writing.

Living Will
A living will tells your health-care professional whether you want death-delaying procedures used if you have a terminal condition and are unable to state your wishes. A living will, unlike a health care power of attorney, only applies if you have a terminal condition. A terminal condition means an incurable and irreversible condition such that death is imminent and the application of any death delaying procedures serves only to prolong the dying process.
Even if you sign a living will, food and water cannot be withdrawn if it would be the only cause of death. Also, if you are pregnant and your health-care professional thinks you could have a live birth, your living will cannot go into effect.
You can use a standard living will form or write your own. You may write specific directions about the death-delaying procedures you do or do not want.
Two people must witness your signing of the living will. Your health-care professional cannot be a witness. It is your responsibility to tell your health-care professional if you have a living will if you are able to do so. You can cancel your living will at any time, either by telling someone or by canceling it in writing.
If you have both a health care power of attorney and a living will, the agent you name in your power of attorney will make your health-care decisions unless he or she is unavailable.

Mental Health Treatment Preference Declaration
A mental health treatment preference declaration lets you say if you want to receive electroconvulsive treatment (ECT) or psychotropic medicine when you have a mental illness and are unable to make these decisions for yourself. It

also allows you to say whether you wish to be admitted to a mental health facility for up to 17 days of treatment.

You can write your wishes and/or choose someone to make your mental health decisions for you. In the declaration, you are called the "principal" and the person you choose is called an "attorney-in-fact." Neither your health-care professional nor any employee of a health-care facility in which you reside may be your attorney-in-fact. Your attorney-in-fact must accept the appointment in writing before he or she can start making decisions regarding your mental health treatment. The attorney-in-fact must make decisions consistent with any desires you express in your declaration unless a court orders differently or an emergency threatens your life or health.

Your mental health treatment preference declaration expires three years from the date you sign it. Two people must witness you signing the declaration. The following people may not witness your signing of the declaration: your health-care professional; an employee of a health-care facility in which you reside; or a family member related by blood, marriage or adoption. You may cancel your declaration in writing prior to its expiration as long as you are not receiving mental health treatment at the time of cancellation. If you are receiving mental health treatment, your declaration will not expire and you may not cancel it until the treatment is successfully completed.

Do-Not-Resuscitate Order
You may also ask your health-care professional about a do-not-resuscitate order (DNR order). A DNR order is a medical treatment order stating that cardiopulmonary resuscitation (CPR) will not be attempted if your heart and/or breathing stops. The law authorizing the development of the form specifies that an individual (or his or her authorized legal representative) may execute the IDPH Uniform DNR Advance Directive directing that resuscitation efforts shall not be attempted. Therefore, a DNR order completed on the IDPH Uniform DNR Advance Directive contains an advance directive made by an individual (or legal representative), and also contains a physician's order that requires a physician's signature.

Before a DNR order may be entered into your medical record, either you or another person (your legal guardian, health care power of attorney or surrogate decision maker) must consent to the DNR order. This consent must be witnessed by two people who are 18 years or older. If a DNR order is entered into your medical record, appropriate medical treatment other than CPR will be given to you. This webpage provides a copy of the Illinois Department of Public Health (IDPH) Uniform Do Not Resuscitate (DNR) Advance Directive that may be used by you and your physician. This webpage also provides a link to guidance for individuals, health-care professionals and health-care providers concerning the IDPH Uniform DNR Advance Directive.

What happens if you don't have an advance directive?
Under Illinois law, a health care "surrogate" may be chosen for you if you cannot make health-care decisions for yourself and do not have an advance directive. A health care surrogate will be one of the following persons (in order of priority): guardian of the person, spouse, any adult child(ren), either parent, any adult brother or sister, any adult grandchild(ren), a close friend, or guardian of the estate.

The surrogate can make all health-care decisions for you, with certain exceptions. A health care surrogate cannot tell your health-care professional to withdraw or withhold life-sustaining treatment unless you have a "qualifying condition," which is a terminal condition, permanent unconsciousness, or an incurable or irreversible condition. A "terminal condition" is an incurable or irreversible injury for which there is no reasonable prospect of cure or recovery, death is imminent and life-sustaining treatment will only prolong the dying process. "Permanent unconsciousness" means a condition that, to a high degree of medical certainty, will last permanently, without improvement; there is no thought, purposeful social interaction or sensory awareness present; and providing life-sustaining treatment will only have minimal medical benefit. An "incurable or irreversible condition" means an illness or injury for which there is no reasonable prospect for cure or recovery, that ultimately will cause the patient's death, that imposes severe pain or an inhumane burden on the patient, and for which life-sustaining treatment will have minimal medical benefit.

Two doctors must certify that you cannot make decisions and have a qualifying condition in order to withdraw or withhold life-sustaining treatment. If your health care surrogate decision maker decides to withdraw or withhold life-sustaining treatment, this decision must be witnessed by a person who is 18 years or older. A health care surrogate may consent to a DNR order, however, this consent must be witnessed by two individuals 18 years or older. A health care surrogate, other than a court-appointed guardian, cannot consent to certain mental health treatments, including treatment by electroconvulsive therapy (ECT), psychotropic medication or admission to a mental health facility. A health care surrogate can petition a court to allow these mental health services.

Final Notes
You should talk with your family, your health-care professional, your attorney, and any agent or attorney-in-fact that you appoint about your decision to make one or more advance directives or a DNR order. If they know what health care you want, they will find it easier to follow your wishes. If you cancel or change an advance directive or a DNR order in the future, remember to tell these same people about the change or cancellation.

125

No health-care facility, health-care professional or insurer can make you execute an advance directive or DNR Order as a condition of providing treatment or insurance. It is entirely your decision. If a health-care facility, health-care professional or insurer objects to following your advance directive or DNR order then they must tell you or the individual responsible for making your health-care decisions. They must continue to provide care until you or your decision maker can transfer you to another health-care provider who will follow your advance directive or DNR order.

Illinois Department of Health
http://www.idph.state.il.us/public/books/advdir4.htm
Retrieved April 5, 2010.

[4]From Chapter Thirteen

Barry Reisberg, M.D., Clinical Director of the New York University School of Medicine's Silberstein Aging and Dementia Research Center first suggested the stages of Alzheimer's disease. The following is excerpted from information available from the Alzheimer's Association, Aging Home Health Care, and other online resources.

Stage 1: No impairment
Stage 2: Very mild cognitive decline (may be normal age-related changes or earliest signs of Alzheimer's disease)
Individuals may feel as if they have memory loss and lapses.
Stage 3: Mild cognitive decline
Friends, family or co-workers begin to notice deficiencies. Common difficulties include:
-Word- or name-finding problems noticeable to family or close associates
-Losing or misplacing a valuable object
Stage 4: Moderate cognitive decline
At this stage, a careful medical interview detects clear-cut deficiencies.
-Impaired ability to perform challenging mental arithmetic-for example, to count backward from 75 by 7s
-The affected individual may seem subdued and withdrawn, especially in socially or mentally challenging situations
Stage 5: Moderately severe cognitive decline
Major gaps in memory and deficits in cognitive function emerge. Some assistance with day-to-day activities becomes essential.
Stage 6: Severe cognitive decline
Memory difficulties continue to worsen, significant personality changes may emerge and affected individuals need extensive help with customary daily activities.
Stage 7: Very severe cognitive decline
This is the final stage of the disease when individuals lose the ability to respond to their environment, the ability to speak and, ultimately, the ability to control movement.

Alzheimer's Association

http://www.alz.org/alzheimers_disease_stages_of_alzheimers.asp
Retrieved June 2, 2010.

Also available from Aging Home Health Care
http://www.aginghomehealthcare.com/stages-of-alzheimers.html
Retrieved September 1, 2010.

www.ingramcontent.com/pod-product-compliance
Lightning Source LLC
Chambersburg PA
CBHW020526290526
45786CB00002B/770